CARING FOR YOUR OLDER
CAT

Chris C. Pinney, D.V.M.

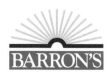

BARRON'S

Dedication

To Tracy, Alexandra, Hunter, and Dakota

All inquiries should be addressed to:
Barron's Educational Series, Inc.
250 Wireless Boulevard
Hauppauge, New York 11788

Library of Congress Catalog Card No. 95-25360

International Standard Book No. 0-8120-9148-5

Library of Congress Cataloging-in-Publication Data
Pinney, Chris C.
  Caring for your older cat / by Chris C. Pinney.
    p.   cm.
  Includes index.
  ISBN 0-8120-9148-5
  1. Cats. 2. Cats—Aging. 3. Cats—Health.
4. Cats—Diseases. 5. Veterinary geriatrics.
I. Title.
SF447.P56   1996
636.8′089897—dc20   95-25360
                                        CIP

Printed in Hong Kong

6789   9955   987654321

Acknowledgments

The author would like to thank M. D. Willard, D.V.M., MS, Diplomate ACVIM, and the College of Veterinary Medicine, Texas A&M University, and Gary Norsworthy, D.V.M., for their valuable contributions to this book.

About the Author

Chris C. Pinney, D.V.M., has written numerous books and articles about health care for pets, including Barron's *Guide To Home Pet Grooming* and *Caring For Your Older Dog*. He has also hosted television and radio shows spotlighting pets and veterinary medicine. He continues to practice small animal medicine, with an emphasis on preventive and emergency care. He resides with his wife and three children in Schulenburg, Texas.

Photo Credits

The majority of the photographs in this book were taken by M. D. Willard, D.V.M. and the Biomedical Learning Resource Center, College of Veterinary Medicine, Texas A&M University. The photographs appearing on the following pages were taken by the author: 30, 31, 33, 36, 75, 88, 94, 187, and inside front cover; Dennis Dunleavy: 139; Bonnie Nance: viii, 4, 8, 34 (top right), 179, 190, front and back covers, and inside back cover; Gary Norsworthy, D.V.M.: 1, 2, 12, 27, 28, 32, 34 (bottom left), 48, 52, 57, 58, 68, 87, 99, 100, 113, 128, 136, 138, 158, 182, 185, 186.

Important Note

Always use caution and common sense whenever handling a cat, especially one that may be ill or injured. Employ proper restraint devices as necessary. In addition, if the information and procedures contained in this book differ in any way from your veterinarian's recommendations concerning your pet's health care, please consult him/her prior to their implementation. Finally, because each individual pet is unique, always consult your veterinarian before administering any type of treatment or medication to your pet.

Contents

Preface

Welcome to *Caring for Your Older Cat*. In your hands you hold an important tool for enhancing the longevity and lifestyle of your elderly feline companion. With recent advancements in veterinary medicine and increased owner attention to preventive health care, cats today are living longer than ever! By learning and applying the information contained in *Caring for Your Older Cat*, you can play a positive, active role in enriching the relationship you share with your pet.

Caring for Your Older Cat is chock-full of information on elderly cats and how to keep them healthy. Chapters One and Two begin with studies on the factors that determine longevity in cats, as well as the effects that aging has upon the various biological systems within the body. Preventive health care is discussed in Chapter Three, with tips on nutrition, exercise, travel, grooming, vaccinations, and parasite control. A special section is even included on sedation and anesthesia in older cats, a subject that can be a source of tension and worry in those owners with pets requiring surgery. Chapter Four is designed to help you better understand and interpret reports and results from diagnostic tests performed on your cat by your veterinarian. Because this is one area in which many pet owners lack sufficient knowledge, this chapter is sure to improve communication and confidence when you discuss test results with your cat's doctor.

Next, *Caring for Your Older Cat* focuses on select diseases and disorders seen in mature felines. In Chapter Five, each biological organ system and associated diseases are presented, as are specific diagnostics and treatments for each condition where applicable. You will learn the latest information on the feline leukemia and feline immunodeficiency viruses, two deadly scourges of cat populations across the country. You will also gain a better understanding of kidney disease and cardiomyopathy, two of the most common afflictions of older felines. Diseases of the respiratory, reproductive, musculoskeletal, nervous, endocrine, and digestive systems are also discussed, as well as the integumentary and immune systems and diseases of the eyes, ears, and nose. Lastly, a comprehensive discussion on neoplasia and cancer is provided to shed light on, among other things, the latest in diagnostics and treatments for the various types of neoplastic conditions that can strike elderly cats.

Chapter Six focuses on clinical signs and symptoms seen in older cats. Handy etiologic listings are included to allow for quick reference, and appropriate courses of action for each are discussed. Keep in mind, though, that these differential listings are meant to be used as guidelines only, and not as substitutes for your veterinarian's sound diagnostic protocols. Remember: The most effective treatment of any disease or disorder begins with a definitive diagnosis!

Would you know what to do if you were confronted with an emergency situation involving your older cat? Chapter Seven offers practical first aid information that could one day save your friend's life.

The final chapter in *Caring for Your Older Cat* deals with euthanasia, a topic that can be uncomfortable at times to discuss. Yet, understanding your pet's final days and what they may entail will help ease the burden of responsibility should a decision ever need to be made. In those instances in which pain and suffering are intense, euthanasia may become the final act of love and kindness you can impart to your old and special friend.

At the back of the book, there is a glossary for reader reference, which defines those terms not commonly known. *Caring for Your Older Cat* is a comprehensive guide designed to improve the quality of life and longevity of your elderly cat and to provide you with loads of veterinary-related information. Details on diseases or disorders not mentioned in this book can be obtained from one or more of the many fine texts dealing with health care for cats available at your favorite bookstore or library. In addition, do not forget to request information concerning issues that pertain to older cats from your veterinarian, who should be more than willing to provide you with such material and answer any questions that may arise.

When properly cared for, cats will provide years of joy and companion-ship.

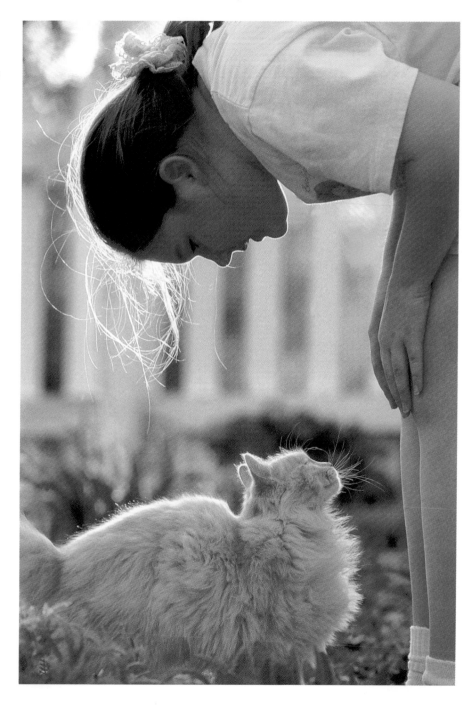

Chapter One
Cats and Longevity

The average life span of a cat is 11 to 15 years, although felines exceeding 20 years of age are becoming more commonplace today. In fact, there is one documented report of a cat that actually reached the ripe old age of 36! What determines how long your feline friend will live? The factors having the most influence on the longevity in your feline companion include genetics, anatomical and physiological considerations, diet, husbandry, and medical care.

Breed type and genetics can certainly influence longevity in cats. For example, of all the different breeds, the Siamese cat seems to have a greater propensity for longevity. On the other hand, Persians tend to have, in general, shorter life spans than do other purebred cats raised under similar environmental conditions. Another genetic factor that can affect the life expectancy of cats is the phenomenon known as "hybrid vigor." Hybrid vigor can occur when two purebred cats of differing breeds are allowed to mate and to produce offspring. Many of these mixed-breed offspring, in turn, exhibit a greater vigor and increased resistance to disease than either of the parents, resulting in a longer life span.

Anatomical and physiological differences between cats can also lead to variations in longevity. For instance, as one might expect, birth defects and other congenital diseases that show up later in life

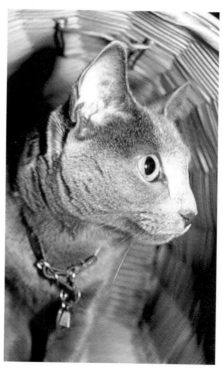

can shorten the life span of an otherwise healthy cat. Inherent differences in metabolic functions and behavior can also cause two cats raised in identical environments to experience different lengths of life. Finally, the inherited competency of the immune system and its ability to respond to disease organisms and conditions as they arise is a major determinant to longevity in felines.

Genetics can exert a strong influence on longevity in cats.

Whereas genetics and other uncontrollable biological factors certainly play a prominent role in

Table 1: Comparison of Ages Between Cats and Humans

Cat	Human
3 months	5 years
6 months	9 years
1 year	15 years
2 years	24 years
3 years	28 years
4 years	32 years
5 years	36 years
6 years	40 years
7 years	44 years
8 years	48 years
9 years	52 years
10 years	56 years
11 years	60 years
12 years	64 years
13 years	68 years
14 years	72 years
15 years	76 years

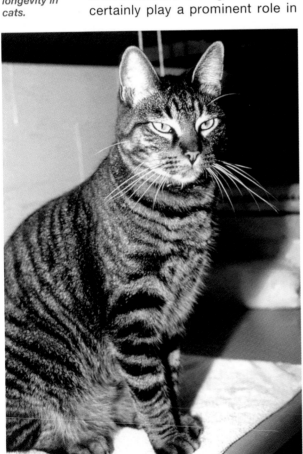

the length of a cat's life, there are a number of other influences that are controllable and can have a significant impact on the feline life span. For example, simply limiting a cat's exposure to environmental dangers such as automobiles, potential poisons, and stray cats that may be harboring the deadly feline leukemia and/or feline immunodeficiency viruses is a major step that can be taken to lengthen the life of a feline pet. Additionally, improved dietary and husbandry protocols and exciting advancements in feline medicine and surgery can add years to the life of a cat. For instance, the development of spe-

**Table 2:
Controllable Factors That
Can Adversely Affect the
Life Span of a Cat**

- Obesity
- Feeding table scraps
- Feeding high-fat, low-fiber diets
- Outdoor roaming
- Lack of attention
- Failure to neuter at a young age
- Failure to vaccinate, especially against FeLV
- Lack of preventive veterinary checkups

cialized rations designed to combat illness in cats, combined with the appearance of newer types of diagnostic tests, medications, and surgical procedures, is helping veterinarians identify and cure diseases that, in the past, would have prematurely ended the life of a pet. Also, increased public awareness of the importance of providing preventive health care, including feeding high-quality diets, providing routine vaccinations, implementing daily grooming sessions, and ensuring regular veterinary checkups, has led to a healthier, and subsequently older, cat population throughout the country.

Chapter Two
The Aging Process and its Effects on Older Cats

Cats age rapidly during the first two years of their lives. With disease, predation, and exposure to the elements adversely affecting the life span of the modern cat's ancestors, the rapid onset of puberty ensured that the species was properly propagated. Following the first two years of life, the aging process slows down, only to again acceler-

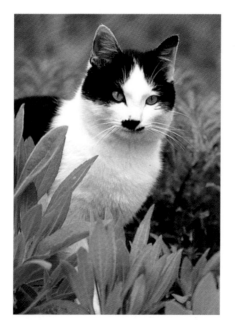

Allowing cats to roam freely outdoors can have an adverse effect on lifespan.

ate as the cat enters into its final years of life. Many of the physical and mental changes associated with aging become readily noticeable during this last trimester of life. A noticeable loss in muscle mass, a slight cloudy and sunken appearance to the eyes, and/or a slight stiffness in the gait are just a few of the changes expected—changes that rarely warrant much ongoing attention from pet owners. However, in addition to these outward signs of aging, it is important to remember that changes are also occurring within the organ systems of the cat's body. And as you may expect, these changes will eventually have an effect on organ function. If not readily recognized and subsequently supported through proper diet and medication, premature organ failure could result, significantly shortening the pet's life. Through regular checkups and appropriate preventive diagnostic tests, your veterinarian can evaluate organ function within your cat's body and determine which, if any, supportive measures are necessary.

Table 3:
General Changes Associated with Aging in Cats

- Dehydration of cells and tissues
- Reduced oxygen flow to tissues
- Decreased ability of cells to maintain their internal environment (homeostasis)
- Reduced immune response
- Declining efficiency of enzyme systems within the body
- Increased incidence of tumor development
- Gradual decline in organ function
- Reduced nervous system responsiveness and personality changes
- Increased susceptibility to stress and decreased adaptability to environmental changes

Aging is the progressive deterioration of metabolic, physiologic, and anatomic structure, function, and efficiency within the body. To begin, the aging process in the cat is marked by a steady decline in the metabolic rate. In a broad sense, *metabolism* refers to the aggregate of all the chemical activities within the body. These chemical reactions both consume energy and produce energy. If the body's metabolic rate is at its normal level, the production

and consumption of energy within the body will be in balance. Imbalances can occur, however, if the rate of metabolism slows, as it does as a cat matures. The effects associated with a slowing metabolism include sluggishness with an increased preponderance toward sleep, a growing intolerance to temperature fluctuations, and rapid tiring after exercise. The immune system also begins to lose its effectiveness with age, creating an increased susceptibility to disease organisms and tumor development. For this reason, older pets must be kept current on their vaccinations. The ability of the body to break down and to eliminate drugs is also reduced with age. As a result, for those pets taking medications for preexisting medical conditions, periodic dosage reviews and adjustments are needed as they mature. Finally, as metabolism slows, caloric needs decline as well. Appropriate dietary adjustments are needed to avoid obesity and other adverse health effects.

With age, it becomes increasingly difficult for the heart to pump blood effectively throughout the body. Furthermore, the blood vessels begin to lose their elasticity. This, combined with a reduced heart output, contributes to a rise in blood pressure, which in turn places even more strain on the geriatric heart. However, restrictions on sodium and fat content, combined with the administration of special medications designed to increase cardiac efficiency and to reduce blood pressure, can be employed to help counteract these aging effects on the feline heart.

As the metabolic rate slows and the blood vessels in the skin become less elastic and lose their ability to dilate and contract in response to temperature fluctuations, temperature intolerance may become noticeable in the older cat. This tends to be magnified by a loss in the skin's insulating ability. Older pets will often seek out the warmth of an owner's lap or the coolness of a bare floor more often than usual. As a result of these *physiological changes*, you should take special care in maintaining relatively constant temperature and humidity within your pet's environment. If elderly cats are allowed to roam outdoors, sweaters and cover-ups designed for cats should be considered if temperatures are below 45°F (7.2°C). On the contrary, when outside temperatures exceed 85°F (29.4°C), it is vital to provide your cat with a generous source of clean, fresh water and, if confined to an outside enclosure, unlimited access to shade.

With increasing age, the capacity of the lungs to provide proper flow and exchange of oxygen to the body decreases. As with reduced heart function, such changes lead to weakness and exercise intolerance. Furthermore, chronic disease and scarring affecting the lung tissue of older cats can also impair blood circulation within the lungs, placing even more burden on an already functionally compromised heart. Behavioral changes, nighttime confusion, and other signs of senility in cats can often be attributed to reduced oxygen flow to the brain caused by poor heart and lung output.

In response to the increased oxygen requirement of an older pet, the air within your pet's environment should be kept fresh, smoke-free, and well circulated. Second-hand smoke can pose a serious health risk to cats suffering from lung conditions. In addition, excess humidity allowed to build up within a cat's environment can adversely affect the rate of oxygen exchange within the lungs. As a result, atmospheric filters and dehumidifiers should be considered in high-humidity areas.

As the digestive system ages, its efficiency at breaking down foodstuffs for absorption into the body is reduced. For starters, periodontal disease (tooth and gum disease) commonly affects older cats and can lead to tooth loss. Routine veterinary dental checkups, combined with at-home dental care, are needed to help slow this progression and to preserve the important digestive function of the teeth. A reduction in salivary secretions in the older pet may lead to a diminished food intake and make swallowing difficult. In many instances, special medications designed to increase the amount of saliva produced and secreted may be needed. The stomach and intestines of older cats become much less tolerant to excesses and dietary fluctuations. Flare-ups of gastritis and colitis can become commonplace and warrant prompt medical attention when they occur to prevent complications. Poor liver and intestinal function in elderly felines can predispose them to constipation. As a result, increased dietary fiber and mild laxatives are often needed. Finally, reduced pancreatic and liver function may decrease with age, interfering with the conversion of foodstuffs to usable nutrients, and making it more difficult for the body to neutralize and eliminate toxic wastes. Again, dietary adjustments made as a cat enters its senior years are the most effective ways to lessen the impact of these age-related consequences.

Within the urinary system, a reduced blood flow to the kidneys and overall age-related wear and tear create scarring and other undesirable changes that disrupt normal blood filtering and waste elimination. Subsequently, toxin and waste buildup within the bloodstream can lead to mental dullness, stomach ulcers, and other disturbances. Feeding elderly felines only high-quality diets and offering a clean (preferably filtered) source of water can help aging kidneys. In addition, good preventive dental care will also help keep bacteria to a minimum.

Reproductive performance and fertility in both the male and the female cat decline with advancing age. Mammary tumors and uterine infections increase in incidence as female cats enter their senior years. Although older male cats don't suffer from diseases and tumors of the prostate and testicles as often as their aged canine counterparts do, they are still at risk. The key to avoiding most reproductive disorders related to aging is to neuter cats, both male and female, at a very young age. If a cat is to be bred, neutering should be performed as soon as its optimum reproductive life is complete (usually around eight years of age) or once the decision is made not to breed the cat any further, whichever comes first.

A decreased blood and oxygen flow to the brain, combined with age-related degeneration of the nervous components of the senses (vision, hearing, smell, and taste) can lead to senile behavioral patterns in cats older than ten years of age. These pets become less and less tolerant to disruptions in normal daily routine as they mature. In addition, reactions to external stimuli become slowed, and as senility sets in further, abnormal behaviors, such as poor recognition of otherwise familiar people and surroundings, poor appetite, and excretory indifference, can result.

As the pet owner you can be supportive of these nervous system changes and sensory deficits in a number of different ways as they occur. For instance, maintaining consistent and recognizable surroundings is important. Invisible fencing devices or physical obstructions can be used to render off-limits certain areas of the house or yard that may prove hazardous. Remembering to approach cats that are visually or mentally impaired slowly and audibly will help prevent startled and/or aggressive reactions. To adjust for diminished senses of smell and taste, rations may be warmed prior to feeding. Finally, increasing your vocal pitch can help compensate for your pet's diminished hearing caused by nerve deafness.

Aging is also accompanied by a degeneration of the endocrine (hormone-producing) glands within the body. *Hormones* are the mediators of many vital processes and reactions occurring within the body, and deficiencies or excesses can lead to a multitude of health problems. To identify any imbalances that may arise as a result of aging, such as hyperthyroidism, diabetes mellitus, and feline endocrine alopecia, routine blood tests designed to assess the various endocrine functions should be performed at least once a year in cats more than eight years of age.

The bones, joints, and muscles, which serve as the support and locomotory system of the body, experience tremendous levels of wear and tear during the normal life of a cat. With aging, cartilage lining the joint surfaces can begin to split and fragment, causing arthritis and joint pain. In addition, a generalized thinning of bone tissue occurs, causing weakness in the cat's overall skeletal structure. Loss of muscle mass and joint flexibility, caused by decreased activity levels, decreased nerve function to the muscles, and excessive protein loss from the body, places even more pressure on the skeletal system. Finally, musculoskeletal disorders caused by age-related disruptions in organ and gland function within

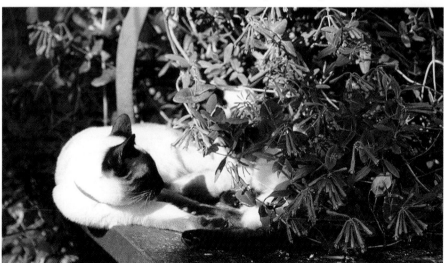

With age comes the need for more sleep and downtime.

the body can materialize. Such disruptions can lead to toxin buildup or hormone-induced changes within the muscle and bone tissue, leading to muscle pain, inflammation, bone thinning, and lameness.

To help alleviate the musculoskeletal effects of aging, elderly cats should be placed on a moderate exercise program to keep their joints limber and muscles toned. Exercise can also help counteract the age-related thinning and brittleness of bone tissue. In addition, routine blood testing performed as a part of an overall preventive health care program can help detect organ or endocrine disturbances.

A generalized thinning of hair, increased susceptibility to infection, and decreases in insulating capabilities are but three of the many changes that can affect the skin and hair coat of cats as they grow older. The skin itself loses its elasticity, with an increase in tissue thickness and dryness. Fluctuations in the rate of skin cell growth and turnover, along with aberrations in the production of oily sebum by the sebaceous glands, can leave the surfaces of the skin and coat of the elderly cat excessively greasy and tacky. Decreased grooming activity that accompanies aging, combined with this oily buildup, can give the hair coat an unkempt, matted appearance, and so older cats should be brushed on a daily basis. Because of decreases in immune system efficiencies and skin changes, older cats also become more susceptible to parasitic inva-

Table 4:
Most Prevalent Causes of Death in Older Cats

- Kidney failure
- Cardiomyopathy
- Cancer
- Physical accidents
- Accidental poisonings
- Feline leukemia-related disease

sion from fleas, ticks, and mites, resulting in special attention to parasite control. Allergies, which can afflict cats of any age, tend to worsen as maturity sets in, and warrant prompt medical attention to prevent secondary skin infections and other associated complications. Finally, hormonal changes or internal organ malfunction caused by aging or by age-related diseases often manifest themselves as skin and hair coat disorders. For this reason, all felines more than six years of age that suffer from such disorders should have blood hormone and enzyme levels tested.

The changes occurring in the body as a result of aging are complex and significant. Many of the conditions can be avoided or their impact lessened by understanding those key points concerning husbandry and preventive health care. By actively applying these concepts and methods, you will positively impact the quality of life of your older cat and ensure that its golden years are filled with health and happiness.

Chapter Three
Preventive Health Care for Older Cats

The old maxim, "An ounce of prevention is worth a pound of cure," is certainly the case when it comes to senior adult cats. A thorough preventive and maintenance health care plan is essential for maintaining a high standard of health and quality of life for your mature pet. Many disease conditions and age-related changes seen in older cats can be slowed or even prevented through the proper implementation of such a program. Important areas in a well-balanced preventive health care program include nutrition and weight management, exercise, vaccinations, internal and external parasite control, regular grooming, dental care, and travel guidelines.

Nutrition for Your Older Cat

Once your pet reaches seven years of age, dietary changes are warranted to accommodate for the effects of aging and the wear and tear on the organ systems of the body. Goals of this senior nutritional program include providing the highest level of nutrition and at the same time maintaining an ideal body weight, slowing the progression of disease and age-related changes, and reducing or eliminating the clinical manifestations of specific disease conditions. For instance, as your cat's metabolic rate slows and the tendency toward obesity increases with advancing age, increasing the amount of fiber and reducing the amount of fat in

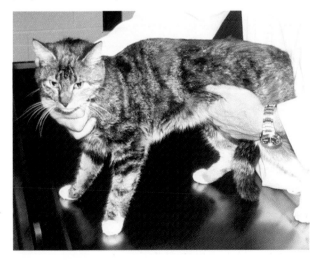

Table 5:
Dietary Management of Disease in Older Cats*

Disease	Dietary Adjustments Recommended
Allergy (food)	Substitute existing protein source in ration with hypoallergenic protein sources such as lamb, rabbit, turkey, or duck
Anemia	High-protein/high-energy diet; multivitamin/mineral supplement
Cachexia	High-protein/high-energy diet; multivitamin/mineral supplement
Colitis	High-fiber balanced diet
Constipation	Low-fat, high-fiber diet
Diabetes mellitus	High-fiber diet
Diarrhea	Low-fiber, low-fat diet
Feline urologic syndrome	Restricted magnesium, high-energy diet; contains ingredients that acidify the urine
Hairballs	Low-fat, high-fiber diet
Heart disease	Restricted sodium diet
Kidney disease	Restricted protein, restricted phosphorus and sodium diet
Liver disease	Restricted protein, low-fat, restricted sodium diet
Obesity	Low-fat, high-fiber diet
Pancreatic insufficiency/ pancreatitis	Low-fiber, low-fat diet
Regurgitation (esophageal disease)	Low-fiber, low-fat, highly digestible diet
Vomiting	Low-fiber, low-fat diet

*Commercially prepared prescription diets are available from your veterinarian and should be used to accomplish the above dietary adjustments.

the diet can help keep the calories at bay and maintain a constant body weight. In addition, as the kidneys begin to lose their ability to handle the waste materials that must be removed from the body, dietary adjustments can play a major role in reducing the amounts of waste products that the kidneys have to process. Simply reducing the sodium content of a ration can exert significant effects in lowering

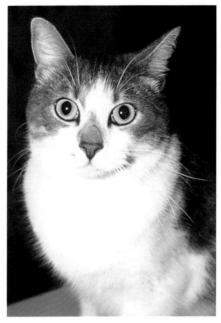

Proper nutrition will help keep your aging cat healthy and youthful in appearance.

blood pressure and reducing the workload placed on an aging heart. Furthermore, increased levels of unsaturated fatty acids and zinc in the diet can help counteract some of the effects that aging has on the skin and hair coat. Finally, because older pets tend to have reduced sensory input (taste and smell), increasing the palatability of the diet can keep even the most finicky senior satisfied.

To summarize, here are some guidelines to follow when it comes to feeding and maintaining an optimum lifestyle for your older cat:

• If your cat is healthy, feed a high-quality ration formulated for the needs of healthy older cats. As cats enter into their senior years, their caloric intake should be maintained at approximately 32 calories per pound of body weight to accommodate changes in metabolism, assuming, of course, that they are not underweight to begin with. To control calories while at the same time satisfying appetite cravings, these "senior" rations typically contain more fiber and less fat than those foods designed for younger cats. Increases in fiber content also serve to promote healthy bowel function in older pets. In addition, any ration fed to your cat should have adequate levels of the amino acid taurine. Deficiencies in this protein building block have been known to cause blindness and cardiomyopathy. Because there are so many brands of senior formulas available on the market today, narrow your choices and ensure proper nutritional balance by asking your veterinarian to recommend the brand that would best suit your cat.

• Those felines suffering from specific illnesses will require special diets prescribed by your veterinarian. For example, cats experiencing constipation, certain types of colitis, chronic hairballs, and diabetes mellitus often require a fiber content in their ration even greater than that found in standard "senior" formulas. In addition, older cats suffering from chronic diarrhea, excessive gas production, and/or pancreatic problems can often benefit from special diets formulated to be more easily digestible than standard fare. Recommended dietary management of cats suffering from heart and/or kidney disease includes diets low in sodium and with restricted levels of protein (not to exceed 28 percent of dry matter). Lastly, older cats that are underweight because of underlying disease may require a diet with increased caloric density to help reestablish their desired weight. Remember: Because all of these prescribed diets are so specialized, be sure to follow your veterinarian's directions closely as to the amounts to feed and frequency of feedings.

- Unless your veterinarian says otherwise, older cats should be fed rations free-choice; that is, they should be allowed unlimited access to their food. Free-choice feeding (versus feeding only one to two times daily) will help ensure that proper amounts are being consumed. In addition, more frequent consumption of smaller amounts of food can aid in the digestive process and nutrient absorption, especially in those cats challenged by age-related changes within the digestive system. In multi-cat households where a dominant cat may prevent others from free-choice feeding, three to four supervised feedings throughout the day can provide a suitable alternative to the free-choice method.
- Vitamin and mineral supplements are rarely required if you are feed-

ing your cat a veterinary-recommended ration. In fact, feeding such a supplement indiscriminately or inappropriately could lead to nutritional imbalances that can have detrimental effects on your pet's health. As a result, do so only under the direct supervision of your veterinarian.

- Implement a regular daily program of moderate exercise for your cat to promote weight control and to enhance digestive processes and normal bowel function.
- Weigh your cat on a monthly basis to detect any significant weight fluctuations. In general, fluctuations greater than 3 pounds (1.4 kg) over a three-month period should warrant attention. Such changes could be indicators of overfeeding, improper diet, or the onset of underlying disease conditions.
- As for feeding table scraps and junk food to your older pet: Don't! It only serves to cause obesity and shorten life spans. If you feel compelled to offer your cat treats during the day, consider using a kibbled form of a senior or low-fat ration. To provide your cat with a satisfying variety, you can even use a brand of food other than the one you are currently feeding. Just remember that even such healthy snacks should account for no more than 5 percent of your pet's total daily caloric intake.
- Always provide your cat with easy access to a source of fresh, clean water. Consumption of proper

amounts of water will help prevent dehydration and encourage frequent urination, which in itself will help decrease the risk of feline urologic syndrome (FUS). Also remember that cats suffering from kidney impairment or endocrine diseases such as diabetes may drink (and require) excessive amounts of water; as a result, be sure that the water bowl never runs dry. (Note: Whenever assessing daily water consumption by a cat, remember that felines fed canned cat food will usually drink less water than those cats on dry rations, because canned foods can have a water content as high as 75 percent!)

The two main causes of obesity in older cats are improper diet and insufficient amounts of exercise.

- Practice good dental hygiene on your cat, including at-home brushing and periodic professional teeth cleaning. Preventing periodontal disease will help keep appetite levels high and ensure proper mastication and preliminary digestion of consumed food.

- Switch to semiannual veterinary checkups to assess your pet's health and to determine whether or not a dietary adjustment or change is warranted. Remember: Feeding the correct diet for your pet's specific needs will lengthen your years of companionship.

Battling Obesity in the Older Cat

Keeping your cat's weight under control is one of the most effective ways to add years to its life. *Obesity* can be defined as an increase in body fat resulting in an increase in body weight more than 10 percent above the normal weight for the cat's breed or body type. Although obese cats aren't candidates for atherosclerosis and subsequent myocardial infarction like an obese human would be, they are predisposed to a variety of other serious disorders such as hypertension, cardiac fatigue, pancreatitis, diabetes mellitus, liver disease, and colitis. Skin disorders seem to be more prevalent in overweight cats, as are disorders of the musculoskeletal and nervous systems. Simply put, obesity reduces the overall quality of life of those unfortunate pets afflicted with it.

The primary causes of obesity in cats are feeding too much food or feeding the wrong types .of food

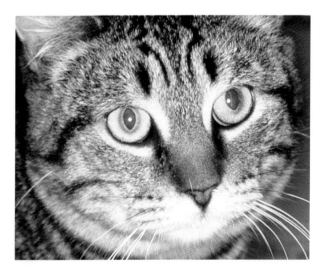

and insufficient amounts of exercise. Failure to adjust dietary requirements and amounts fed based on specific individual needs as a pet matures is a common mistake made by pet owners. To help counteract the effects of a slower metabolic rate, healthy seniors more than seven years of age should be fed "less active" or "senior" diets containing higher fiber and fewer calories instead of the regular adult maintenance rations. Also, senior cats should be fed a diet consisting of one food type only, unless a medical condition stipulates otherwise. Under no circumstances should table scraps be fed to a cat; table scraps promote obesity and lead to finicky eating behaviors.

If your cat is obese, simply cutting back on the amount you feed will not provide the lasting weight loss you desire. In fact, depriving your cat of adequate amounts of food could create a state of malnutrition, leading to incessant begging and self-induced dietary indiscretions. The correct way to achieve weight loss through dietary adjustment is to feed your cat a ration that is specially formulated for weight loss. This kind of diet is readily available from and should be recommended by your veterinarian. It generally contains a high-fiber content, which allows for caloric reduction while satisfying the hunger of your pet. Feed the amount recommended on the bag or can that corresponds to your pet's ideal weight. If you don't know what this should be, consult your veterinarian.

Taurine Deficiencies in Older Cats

Taurine is an essential amino acid in cats; that is, it must be present in a cat's diet because it cannot be synthesized internally. Deficiencies in taurine can lead to severe health consequences, including dilated cardiomyopathy, feline central retinal degeneration and blindness, neurologic disease, and immunosuppression.

Older cats require between 1,000 and 1,500 parts per million of taurine in their diet. This amount should be raised to 2,000 ppm taurine in those cats that are fed moist cat foods. In the past ten years, commercial cat food manufacturers have placed special emphasis on the levels of taurine included in their rations. As a result, dietary-induced taurine deficiencies are rare in today's cats fed quality commercially available cat foods. However, deficiencies in taurine can also be caused by digestive disturbances that interfere with a proper absorption of taurine. For instance, older cats suffering from chronic colitis and inflammatory bowel disease (IBD) have increased susceptibility to taurine deficiencies and subsequent cardiomyopathies. Felines suffering from such chronic digestive disturbances usually require a taurine-rich diet or supplementation to prevent degenerative changes. Taurine supplements in paste or capsule forms are available from veterinarians. Minced clams and tuna also are excellent sources of taurine, but they should not be fed as the sole diet because by themselves they are not nutritionally complete.

Exercise and Your Older Cat

Along with dietary adjustments, exercise is a vital part of any weight control or weight loss program. Implementing a moderate exercise program into the daily routine of your older cat will not only help prevent or combat obesity but will also increase muscle tone and strength and help counteract some of the loss in muscle mass associated with aging. Exercise will improve agility and flexibility and help loosen up stiff joints. In addition, improved blood circulation, heart function, and lung capacities resulting from exercise all serve to increase your pet's quality of life. Regular activity will also promote and improve gastrointestinal motility and increase urination frequency, the latter being an important factor in the prevention of feline urologic syndrome (FUS).

Before you implement any exercise program for your cat, a complete physical exam should be performed by your veterinarian to identify any underlying health conditions that may limit the type and amount of exercise performed. In addition, if the exercise program entails time spent outdoors, it is important that your cat is current on its vaccinations.

Designated daily play sessions and brisk aerobic walks using a leash and harness are the two main methods of ensuring that your cat gets the appropriate amount of healthy exercise. The type of play you engage in with your cat does not matter, as long as you have a willing participant and can keep the level of activity brisk and dynamic. These play sessions should last a minimum of 15 minutes in order to provide for effective calorie burn.

Leash-Training Your Cat

Although it is true that cats can be somewhat independent creatures, they can (and should) be taught to walk on a leash and harness. All that is usually required to leash-train your cat is the correct equipment and a generous portion of patience on your part. A harness specifically designed for cats and a 6- to 8-foot (1.8–2.4 m) leash can be purchased from your local pet supply or veterinary office. Collars and extendable leashes should not be used when walking cats, as both afford very little control.

Begin your training efforts by allowing your cat to wear the harness around the house without the leash attached. If your cat objects when you first apply the harness, leave it on for only a few minutes each day for the first three to five days. From then on, each day gradually increase the amount of time that the harness is left on until its presence becomes second nature to your cat. (Note: Do not allow your cat to wear the harness if allowed to roam free outdoors, for if it became entangled upon a fence post or tree limb, your pet could be seriously injured).

Once your cat becomes accustomed to the harness, begin attaching the leash to the harness during the training sessions and coaxing your cat to walk on lead. Keep initial sessions brief and use only gentle tugs. Don't drag an unwilling subject around the house; this will only serve to make future training difficult. Remember: A major goal of any training program is to make it a pleasant experience. Be sure to praise heavily whenever desired results are achieved instead of punishing for improper responses. Over time you will find that your cat will respond favorably to such training techniques and reward you with results.

After your feline has become used to walking around indoors on the leash and harness, it is time to move the training sessions outdoors. Again, keep the initial sessions short and effective. Cats that have not spent much time outdoors will require days or weeks of adjustment to the new environment. Purposely avoid direct encounters with people and other pets during this introductory period in order to keep stress to a minimum.

Training your cat to walk outdoors on a leash requires patience and persistence on your part. If your cat is out of shape, keep the aerobic exercise sessions short and of low intensity. The ultimate goal is to work up to 15 to 20 minutes of brisk, continuous aerobic walking daily.

Following exercise, provide your cat access to plenty of fresh water to allow for replacement of fluids lost from physical exertion. This is especially important in older felines, because if a cat is suffering from even a mild degree of kidney impairment and cannot replace fluids, dehydration and overt kidney failure could result.

Remain alert for signs of overexertion and/or heart trouble. These signs can include rapid tiring, coughing, and/or breathing difficulties. If you notice such symptoms at any point during the exercise routine, stop immediately. If your cat is not breathing regularly within three to four minutes, contact your veterinarian.

Traveling with Your Older Cat

Older cats have special needs that must be taken into consideration, whenever they are being transported by car or plane, in order to reduce the chances of injury and stress-induced complications. In all cases, the safety and comfort of the passenger (and driver, when applicable) must always be kept in mind first and foremost. You as a responsible pet owner can help achieve these goals by following a few basic travel guidelines.

When transporting an older cat by automobile, a travel carrier must be used. Not only will your pet feel more secure in a carrier, helping to reduce stress associated with the ride, but the carrier will help minimize jostling and jolting movements that could prove quite painful to older cats with arthritic joints. In addition, be sure to keep the inside of your car well vented and at an air-conditioned temperature between 70 and 80°F (21.1–26.7°C). Excited or stressed felines forced to travel in hot, stuffy car interiors, or cars filled with cigarette or cigar smoke, are likely to suffer ill effects. Cigarette smoke in itself can be quite irritating to the eyes, nose, and mucous membranes of the older cat, and even dangerous to those seniors suffering from heart and/or lung disease. As a courtesy to your feline friend, refrain from smoking until you have reached your destination. Car exhaust fumes can have the same effect as cigarette smoke. If stopped in traffic for any appreciable amount of time, be sure to crack the car windows and keep the air within the car circulating continuously.

As you have heard time and time again, never leave a pet in a parked car unattended for more than five minutes on days when temperatures exceed 72°F (22.2°C) or drop below 55°F (12.8°C). Keep in mind that older pets lose some of their ability to regulate body temperatures effectively in response to temperature fluctuations. As a result, they are more susceptible to heat stroke or hypothermia if left unattended in such conditions. If you do have to leave your pet for a few minutes, be sure to leave two or more windows partially opened to allow for air circulation. In addition, the use of window shields and sun visors is strongly recommended.

For lengthy trips be sure to take along plenty of water, preferably filtered, for your cat to drink. Tip: Consider freezing some water in a bowl prior to the trip to provide a lasting and refreshing source of water. Also plan on frequent stops to allow your cat to leave the carrier and to stretch in the car or outdoors on a leash and harness. Litter boxes or pans can be provided for convenience during stops. Because many cats will refuse to use a litter box on trips, consider lining the bottom of the carrier with an absorbent towel or mat in case accidents happen.

If your cat is prone to motion sickness, try feeding your pet a small amount of food about 30 minutes prior to your trip. Often, an empty stomach coupled with stress can cause motion sickness. Never give your aging pet any medication for anxiety or motion sickness unless it was specifically prescribed by your veterinarian. Tranquilizers

Table 6:
Recommended Annual Vaccinations for Older Cats

Vaccine	Route(s) of Administration*
FVRCP (feline viral rhinotracheitis-calicivirus-panleukopenia)	SQ, IM, IN
FeLV (feline leukemia)	SQ, IM
Rabies	SQ, IM
Feline chlamydia (optional)	SQ, IM
FIP (feline infectious peritonitis) (optional)	IN

*Route of administration dependent upon the type and brand of vaccine administered (SQ = Subcutaneous; IM = Intramuscular; IN = Intranasal)

and antihistamines, two common classes of drugs used for these purposes, can be harmful if given to a pet with an undiagnosed medical condition.

During overnight stays at hotels, it is best to keep your cat confined to the carrier until it is time to retire for the night. Cats experiencing stress that are allowed to roam free within a strange room will often dash for an opened door, or they may find a hole or opening in a hotel room that could prove unaccessible by you. Once you are ready for bed, you can place your cat in the bathroom with a litter box, food bowl, and water bowl. Just be sure to scan the bathroom first for any possible cracks, crevices, or holes that an industrious cat could use to escape.

If you are planning to transport your elderly pet by airplane, extreme caution should be taken. Always consult your veterinarian beforehand to determine whether or not any medical conditions your pet may have could be worsened by such a trip. For example, high altitude flying could be harmful to a cat suffering from heart and/or lung disease. In addition, aged cats that are forced to travel in cargo holds could be adversely affected by temperature and pressure fluctuations. Speak with your airline representatives concerning their accommodations for traveling pets. If at all possible, ask to transport your older cat in a carrier in the passenger compartment.

Regardless of the mode of transportation, be certain to carry copies of your cat's medical record with you when traveling out of town, and find the location of an emergency veterinary hospital where you are staying. If your cat should become ill during your trip, valuable time can be spared if such a location is known in advance. Local phone books will contain such information.

Vaccinations Against Infectious Diseases

The immune system is a complex network of cells, organs, chemicals, and other molecules designed to protect the body against foreign invaders. One method of keeping this system primed for defensive action is through the use of vaccines. Vaccines are composed of one or more *antigens*, substances recognized as foreign by the body and capable of eliciting an immune response. The particular antigens used in the development of feline vaccines include specific viruses and bacteria that have been scientifically altered in such a way as to eliminate their ability to cause disease upon their introduction into a host. However, upon introduction, they will still stimulate special immune cells within the body, called *B lymphocytes*, to produce specific proteins called *antibodies*. These antibodies, in turn, interact with and attach to the foreign invaders, marking them for destruction by other immune cells and chemicals within the body.

There are basically three types of vaccines used in veterinary medicine. *Killed* (inactivated) *vaccines* contain disease entities that have been artificially processed and rendered noninfectious. *Modified-live* (attenuated) *vaccines* contain disease agents that have been treated so that they cannot produce clinical disease when introduced into the host. Unlike killed vaccines, these agents still have the ability to replicate within the host animal. Because of this feature, modified-live vaccines tend to stimulate a greater immune response than do killed vaccines, but they can cause a vaccine-induced disease if they were poorly manufactured or if the pet's immune system is severely depressed. *Subunit vaccines*, which consist of portions or pieces of actual disease agents that are noninfectious in nature, have the ability to stimulate an effective immune response. The advantage of subunit vaccines is that the immune response generated by the disease particles in the vaccine provides immunity against the actual disease agent itself, thereby eliminating the need for use of the actual infective agent in the preparation.

As your cat matures, the importance of maintaining a current vaccination history cannot be overemphasized. As with other organ systems, the function and efficacy of the feline immune system declines with advancing years. As a result, the immune response mounted against a foreign invader may be slowed or delayed just enough to allow the disease organism to gain a foothold within the body. For this reason, priming the aging immune system with regular annual vaccination boosters is a must to help ensure the fastest reaction time possible.

The diseases your older cat should be vaccinated against yearly include feline panleukopenia, feline viral rhinotracheitis (herpes virus), feline calicivirus, feline leukemia, and rabies. In addition, vaccines against feline chlamydial infections and feline infectious peritonitis may also be recommended by your veterinarian if these diseases are prevalent in your area.

Feline panleukopenia (feline distemper) is a viral disease of cats that causes, among other things, severe gastroenteritis and immunosuppression in infected individuals. Caused by a virus similar to parvovirus disease in dogs, feline panleukopenia can be deadly if contracted by an older cat that is not adequately protected against the organism. Unvaccinated kittens pose the greatest threat of this disease to older cats.

Feline viral rhinotracheitis and *feline calicivirus* infections affect the nasal passages and upper airways, causing sneezing, loss of appetite, eye infections, oral ulcers, and nasal discharges. In severe instances, life-threatening pneumonia can result. Vaccines for both conditions are usually combined with the panleukopenia vaccine into a single-dosage vaccine commonly referred to as the FVRCP (feline viral rhino-tracheitis-calicivirus-panleukopenia) vaccine. The FVRCP vaccine is quite effective at preventing all three of these clinical diseases.

Feline leukemia is one of the most important infectious diseases affecting cats today. Caused by the same family of viruses that causes AIDS in humans, feline leukemia can decimate the immune system of infected felines, opening the door to a wide variety of infectious diseases, tumors, and other disease conditions. A number of different vaccines are commercially available against the feline leukemia virus, and one should be administered annually to all cats (following an initial booster series) to help protect them against this disease.

Rabies is certainly the most notorious of all diseases warranting vaccination. Characterized by hydrophobia (fear of water) and other symptoms associated with nervous system disease, such as seizures or paralysis, rabies is uniformly fatal to its unfortunate victims. The incidence of this disease among cats has been steadily rising each year, primarily because of the nocturnal roaming habits of cats (thereby increasing their chances of exposure to a rabid animal) and to owner non-compliance with vaccination recommendations. In cats, rabies is most often transmitted via saliva through a bite wound inflicted by a rabid animal, including other cats, dogs, bats, skunks, and a wide variety of additional wildlife. A conclusive diagnosis of rabies can only be achieved through the microscopic examination of brain tissue from a deceased animal. Because of the potential threat to human health, most states require by law that a rabies vaccination booster be given to all cats on a yearly basis. (Note: Some states only require a booster every three years; however, because of the serious nature of this disease, this author recommends yearly vaccination.) To be legal, all rabies vaccinations must be administered by licensed veterinarians.

Optional vaccines that may be recommended by your veterinarian if the disease incidence is high in your particular area are the *feline chlamydial infection* vaccine and the *feline infectious peritonitis* vaccine. The feline chlaymdia organism can cause a condition in cats known as *feline pneumonitis*. This disease is characterized by intense inflammation within the respiratory airways and lungs, leading to coughing, sneezing, discharges, and breathing difficulties. It can also infect the eyes of cats, causing conjunctivitis and ulcers. Feline

infectious peritonitis is a uniformly fatal disease of cats that can affect organ systems throughout the body. It is usually spread from cat to cat by exposure to infected respiratory droplets. A newer vaccine against this disease is designed to be given as drops in the nose in an effort to stimulate local immunity that would eliminate the organism before it even gained entrance into the body.

Note: To ensure that the vaccinations are administered properly and safely and that the vaccines being used have been stored and handled properly, utilize only the services of a licensed veterinarian when immunizing your cat. The health benefits to your pet and the peace of mind you will have by doing so are well worth the extra cost!

Internal Parasite Control

To ensure that your elderly cat remains free of internal parasites such as roundworms, hookworms, tapeworms, lungworms, and protozoa, a stool check should be performed at least once a year (ideally every six months) by your veterinarian. Early detection and treatment of parasitic infestations will help prevent malnutrition, diarrhea, and stress-related immune system suppression from becoming established and complicating any preexisting medical conditions. It will also

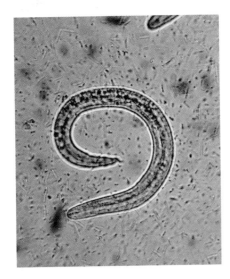

Internal parasite control is a vital part of any preventive health care program for older cats.

lessen the risk of human exposure to these parasites, some of which (roundworms, protozoa) can pose a significant health risk to people, especially children.

Environmental management and cleanliness also plays a key role in the prevention of all internal parasites. For instance, because fleas are the most common carrier of cat tapeworms, rigid flea control measures are essential to protect your cat against infestation by this type of worm. Furthermore, by cleaning the litter box on a daily basis and disposing of any fecal material left in your yard by stray cats, transmission of infective parasite eggs to your pet and to others will be effectively blocked. (For more information on the treatment and prevention on internal parasites, see Internal Parasitism, page 66.)

External Parasite Control

Fleas are the most common external parasites with which your older cat will have to contend. Not only can their bites produce extreme discomfort and even allergic reactions, fleas are also host to the most common tapeworm that affects cats, *Dipylidium caninum*. Aging felines can be particularly tormented by these pests, which may reside on skin regions that an older cat is unable to bite or scratch due to age-related inflexibility or arthritis. Furthermore, maturing cats that are

debilitated by diseases such as kidney failure seem to also be prime targets for fleas. The exact mechanism for this is unknown; however, some feel that changes in internal body chemistries due to disease or aging, or abnormalities in oily secretions from the skin, may be to blame. Regardless of the cause, flea control is a vital part of any preventive health care program implemented on behalf of your older pet.

The key to implementing an effective flea control program is to first acquaint yourself with the lifestyle of this parasite. This life cycle begins with the deposition of eggs both on the host pet and in the pet's environment, including both the house and yard. Those eggs laid on the skin and hair coat of the host will usually fall off into the environment soon after deposition. Within a house, fleas will directly deposit their eggs onto carpeted areas of the home. Other favorite sites include cracks and corners within the house, damp floorboards and cupboards, and even within air-conditioning ducts. Of course, your pet's sleeping quarters will have its fair share of eggs as well. The adult flea will lay 3 to 18 eggs per laying, and in her life span of a year, she may lay over 200 eggs! The rate of this egg laying will increase proportionally with environmental temperature and humidity, and with the numbers of blood meals and male fleas available. Maturity of the eggs occurs most rapidly when the temperature is between 65 and 95°F (18.3–35°C) and the relative humidity is between 50 and 99 percent. In optimum conditions, the eggs hatch into larvae 2 to 14 days after being laid. The small white larvae that emerge from the eggs rely on adult flea excrement for food as they grow. Six months and three molts later, the larvae spin cocoons, in which they remain anywhere from one week to one year. It is important to note that while in this cocoon, these larvae are very resistant to chemical insecticides and other environmental treatment modalities. Once fully mature adult fleas emerge from the cocoon, they diligently search out hosts upon which to feed. Incredibly, the average adult flea can live up to 58 days without food. Some species, after engorging on a blood meal, can live 200 days without another meal.

Unless in the process of feeding, fleas will spend most of their time off your pet and in the environment, in your house or yard. Don't make the mistake of immediately discounting fleas as the cause of your cat's scratching just because you fail to observe a live specimen on the skin. Instead, suspect fleas whenever there is visible chewing activity and hair loss around your cat 's hind legs and the back, especially near the base of the tail. If you part the hair in these areas, you will often see the tiny black flecks of flea excrement that are left behind after feeding. This is a sure sign that you do indeed have visitors.

Because fleas do spend so much of their time off your pet, thorough environmental treatment is necessary. Consultation with your veterinarian is advised when choosing among the many flea remedies and protocols that are safe and effective for your specific needs.

Environmental Treatment for Fleas

To begin, vacuum the carpets and floors of your house, as well as your cat's sleeping quarters, to physically remove as many eggs, cocoons, larvae, and adults as possible. Be sure to dispose of the vacuum bag afterward, because it will contain live fleas or flea larvae that could reinfest the environment through the vacuum cleaner if left in the bag. If a nondisposable bag is used, mothballs kept in the bag will kill any larvae or fleas collected. Next, after removing all people and pets, have your house exterminated, either by hiring a professional exterminator or by spraying, dusting, or using a concentrated fogger containing an approved insecticide yourself. Use an insecticidal product that contains within its ingredient statement an insect growth regulator (IGR) such as methoprene or fenoxycarb. (You may first want to check into whether or not your state has any restrictions on the use of IGRs.) The combination of insecticide and growth regulator will eliminate not only adult fleas, but many of the larval forms as well.

Unless your older cat is kept exclusively indoors, the yard should be treated at the same time as the house with any one of several products approved for this purpose. Chemicals most commonly used for this purpose include chlorpyrifos, malathion, and diazinon. Furthermore, use or request products that are "microencapsulated" or contain ultraviolet light-resistant insect growth regulators (such as fenoxycarb) for greater residual killing activity. For yards, sprays or granules should be used. Treatment of both the house and yard using traditional insecticides should be repeated in 14 days, then again every three to four weeks during flea season to maintain flea-free premises.

In recent years, two notable advancements have been made in the battle against fleas in the environment. The first is the introduction of polymerized borate compounds, available under various brand names from your veterinarian or favorite pet supply. Applied to the carpets and baseboards of your home, these compounds have been electrostatically charged and will kill those fleas with which they come in contact. Noticeable results are usually obtained within a week after application. Best of all, this powder is odorless, easy to use, and safe for pets and children (one notable exception is that this, like any powder, should not be used around cats suffering from feline asthma or other respiratory difficulties). Under normal conditions, application of this product must be performed every 6 to 12 months. Carpets must remain dry for continued efficacy; if the carpet becomes damp or is shampooed, reapplication will be necessary.

The second advancement deals with beneficial nematodes as a mode of controlling fleas in the yard. Also available through your veterinarian or feed stores, these microscopic worms, when applied to a yard, begin eating any and every flea larvae they can find! Harmless to grass, pets, and humans, beneficial nematodes are about as natural as you can get when it comes to flea control for your yard. Weather conditions and environmental temperatures will determine how often treatments must be repeated. Be sure to ask your veterinarian for more information regarding this new method of flea control.

Treating Your Pet for Fleas

At the same time that you are treating your house and yard, you need to be treating your pet. There are many different preparations you can use on your cat. These come in the form of sprays and dusts, collars, shampoos and dips, and many other less conventional vehicles. For older cats, the treatment of choice involves the frequent use of sprays or foams. Flea powders may irritate your cat's airways if accidentally inhaled. Flea collars rarely afford any measure of flea control by themselves, and may prove to be sensitive to the skin of older pets. The two biggest advantages to using approved flea sprays or foams on your cat are safety and the ability to reapply frequently. These products can either be alcohol-based, which provides quick knockdown power against fleas, or they can be water-based for those cats with sensitive skin. In addition, the spray or foam you choose should contain pyrethrins, potentiated pyrethrins, or pyrethroids (resmethrin, permethrin, d-transallethrin, fenvalerate) as the active ingredients. These chemicals are preferred over the stronger, more toxic insecticides, such as organophosphates (chlorpyrifos, dichlorvos) or carbamates (carbaryl), due to their safety and efficacy if utilized properly. Traditionally, the biggest disadvantage in using pyrethrin type products was poor residual flea-fighting activity. However, with the development of "slow-release microencapsulation" technology, the residual activity of these products, and subsequent efficacy, has been dramatically improved. Whenever pyrethrin products are used, frequent application is imperative for effective flea control. In some instances, this must be done on a daily basis. When employing sprays, the most tolerated method of accomplishing their application is to spray a generous amount of the product on a towel or washcloth, then massage it into the hair coat all the way down

to the skin. Excessive salivation immediately following application may occur as a normal feline reaction to anything foreign placed on the hair coat, but this drooling should last only a few minutes. If it lasts over ten minutes, contact your veterinarian. Just be certain that whenever using any insecticidal products on cats, always follow label directions regarding frequencies and methods of application, and note any precautionary statements that may apply.

In addition to flea sprays and foams, shampoos containing an insecticide may also be applied to your pet every two to four weeks to help control fleas. Shampoos containing pyrethrins or pyrethrin derivatives are the safest to use in older cats. Remember, however, that shampooing your cat more than once every two weeks can lead to excessively dry skin, so use only on your veterinarian's recommendation. Flea dips are nothing more than highly concentrated preparations of insecticides. However, because of the high potential for toxicity in felines, alternate methods of treating fleas on your cat should be used before considering insecticidal dips. In most instances, stringent environmental control, combined with frequent application of a flea spray or foam safe for cats, is all that is required to achieve effective flea control.

Apart from the chemicals and preparations already mentioned, countless natural remedies for flea control have been touted as effective alternatives to insecticides. For instance, many pet owners across the country contend that products like brewer's yeast and garlic, when taken in tablet form, are effective at keeping fleas off pets. Unfortunately, controlled scientific studies indicate that little to no flea control benefit is offered by these products. In addition, certain natural products containing abrasive type ingredients (silica gel, diatomaceous earth) have been applied to the skin and coat of some pets in a natural attempt at flea control. However, such substances may dry or irritate your pet's skin, and their effectiveness is also questionable. Finally, although many manufacturers and some pet owners will stand by the effectiveness of electronic flea collars, research has demonstrated that, like other natural remedies, their overall impact in controlling fleas is minimal.

Ear Mites, Ticks, and Mange Mites in Cats

Besides fleas, the next most prevalent external parasite affecting cats is the ear mite. Ear mites are tiny organisms that reside within the external ear canals of cats, causing inflammation, irritation, and a characteristic discharge. This discharge is black and crusty in appearance, and normally involves both ears at the same time. Affected felines will often shake their head and scratch at their ears incessantly in response to the infes-

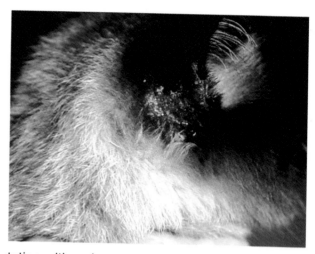

tation, although some may show no such signs. Hairless patches and areas of raw skin below both ears may be seen as a result of these scratching efforts.

Ear mites are highly contagious from cat to cat. Older cats are most likely to become infested by contact with a new kitten brought into a household, or by interaction with other neighborhood cats. As far as multi-pet households are concerned, it is safe to assume that if one pet is diagnosed with ear mites, then all are affected.

Treating ear mites in cats involves the application of an antimite medication (miticide) to both ear canals on a daily basis for 7 to 14 days. These can be purchased as over-the-counter medications at your pet store, or more potent formulations may be obtained from your veterinarian. To improve the efficacy of the treatment, both ears should be thoroughly cleaned with a commercially

Self-trauma secondary to ear mite infestation.

available ear cleanser prior to using the miticidal medication. In addition, to help prevent recurrences, a flea spray or foam should be applied to the cat's hair coat and bedding every four days during the treatment cycle. This will effectively eliminate any mites that may be temporarily residing in these areas.

Due to the grooming habits of cats, tick infestations rarely occur in felines. When found, these unsightly parasites, which attach themselves to their host via sucking mouthparts, are usually located on the head, neck, and ear regions of the cat. In especially severe infestations that remain untreated, marked skin irritation and anemia caused by blood loss can result.

Female ticks lay their eggs in and under sheltered areas in the environment, such as wood stumps, rocks, and wall crevices. Once hatched, the larvae, called "seed ticks," will crawl up onto grass

stems or bushes and attach themselves to a host animal that may pass by. Depending on their life cycle, immature ticks may seek out one to three different host animals to complete the maturation process into an adult.

Because ticks and fleas are sensitive to the same type of chemicals, treatment and control is basically the same. A thorough and consistent treatment of the yard and, if needed, house, with an approved insecticide is the cornerstone of an effective control program. Because ticks can live for months in their surrounding habitat without a blood meal, treatment should be performed every two to four weeks (as with fleas) during the peak flea and tick seasons in your area. For treating your older cat, use a pyrethrin spray to kill any existing ticks attached to the skin and to discourage others from attaching. Never attempt to remove ticks from your cat by applying manual pressure alone, or by applying a hot match or needle to the tick's body. Most ticks killed by the application of a pyrethrin spray will fall off with time once they die. In some cases, you may need to manually remove the dead tick after spraying. When picking them off your cat, use a pair of gloves (because ticks can carry a number of human diseases) and tweezers to grasp the dead tick as close to its attachment site as possible, then pull straight up and away using constant tension. Once the tick is

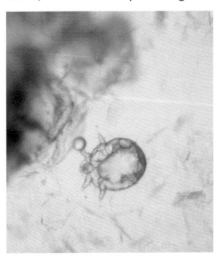

Mite

freed, wash the bite wound with soap and water and then apply a first aid cream or ointment to prevent infection. Again, be sure the tick is completely dead before removal; this will ensure that the tick's mouthparts come out attached to the rest of the body. If left behind, the mouthparts can cause an irritating localized skin reaction.

Mange mites are microscopic parasites belonging to the same zoological class as spiders. Infestations with mange mites are relatively rare in cats, yet may arise following exposure to stray animals or secondary to immune compromise. Living and feeding within the skin or hair follicles of their host, their presence often leads to intense itching, hair loss, and secondary skin infections in affected animals. There are several types of mites that can infest cats, the two most important being *Notoedres cati* and the demodectic mange mite.

For those older cats that are groomed regularly and are not allowed to roam the neighborhood, notoedric mange is rarely a problem. This type of mange mite burrows into the skin and deposits eggs into these tunnels, where the development of the immature mite takes place. Clinical signs seen with notoedric mange are hallmarked by intense itching, hair loss, and/or thickened skin, especially around the ears and neck.

On the contrary, the demodectic mange mite does not burrow, but rather resides within the hair follicles of affected cats. This mange mite usually causes no clinical signs in those cats that have healthy, active immune systems. However, in those cats that may suffer from immunosuppression caused by drug therapy or by certain disease conditions like diabetes mellitus, FeLV (feline leukemia), or FIV (feline immunodeficiency virus), the *Demodex* mange mites may begin to multiply within the hair follicles and produce clinical disease. Symptoms include scattered hair loss and skin scaling, especially around the head, ears, and neck. Itching is usually not a prominent clinical sign unless secondary bacterial infections within the hair follicles are present.

Diagnosis of mange can be made by your veterinarian by observing clinical signs and by examining microscopically scrapings of skin obtained from your cat. Treatment for either type of mange employs the use of special dips and medications designed to kill the mites, and antibiotics if a secondary skin infection is present. In the case of *Demodex*, the cause of the underlying immunosuppression must be addressed as well.

Grooming Your Older Cat

An important part of any preventive health care program is grooming. Not only will it help keep your

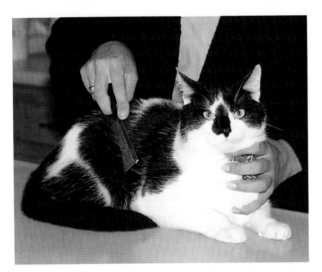

Daily grooming will help keep the hair coat healthy and shiny.

ing with such regular frequency will assist your cat's grooming efforts and help prevent tangles and mats from forming. In addition, it will help remove dead hair from the coat, paving the way for new hair growth and reducing the incidence of hair balls. Brushing also stimulates sebaceous gland activity and blood circulation to the skin, and helps remove skin scales and crusts that could lead to itching in cats, especially those suffering from allergic skin disease.

Bristle brushes work well on the feline coat; as a general rule, the wider apart the bristles are placed on the brush, the longer the coat it is designed to be used on. Combs can also come in quite handy, especially if your cat has a fine, silky hair coat that may be too delicate for conventional brushes. Rubber curry combs, similar to those used on horses, are also recommended for cats, especially those that normally object to conventional brushing. These combs, especially those designed with soft rubber tips, provide the added benefit of giving your cat a gentle massage, making the combing process a pleasant experience.

When brushing or combing, follow the grain of the hair, using firm, even strokes. If you run into a mat or tangle (rare in cats), use your fingers to work as much of it free as you can, then gently run the brush or comb through it. If the mat fails to give way and your pet is experiencing discomfort as a result, stop

cat in top shape physically, but the time spent with your old friend will provide the psychological comfort that such interaction and attention creates. As an added benefit, routine grooming and hands-on attention will assist in the early detection of external parasites, tumors, infections, or any other changes or abnormalities that may result from the germination of an internal disease condition. The grooming program for your older cat should include skin and coat care, nail care, ear care, and dental care.

Brushing and Bathing

Regardless of the hair length of your cat, brushing the hair coat thoroughly on a daily basis will not only promote a healthy coat, but healthy skin as well. In those cats with long hair, twice-a-day brushing may be required, especially during the spring and fall months when shedding occurs the most. Brush-

immediately. Instead, run a comb as close to the skin as possible to entrap the mat on top and then, using scissors, cut the mat at the comb's upper surface. Never leave the skin unprotected when using scissors to remove a mat. Once the mat is finally removed, inspect the skin at that location to be sure it is not reddened or inflamed. If it appears to be only slightly irritated, the condition should resolve on its own now that the mat has been removed. However, if the skin is obviously infected or the area is severely reddened and inflamed, seek veterinary medical attention immediately.

As a rule, cats rarely need to be bathed, especially if you brush your cat on a daily basis. Routine bathing should only be performed on those cats that are continually exposing themselves to excessive dirt, grease, or other noxious substances in their environment, and for those felines suffering from external parasites or medical conditions such as skin infections. If a general cleaning is desired for an otherwise healthy cat, then the best recommendation is to purchase and use a mild hypoallergenic shampoo to use for this purpose. These shampoos are readily available from your veterinarian or favorite pet supply store. If your cat is afflicted with any type of medical condition, then the type of shampoo used should be limited to that recommended or prescribed by your veterinarian.

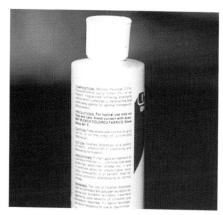

Read all label directions carefully whenever using medicated shampoos and topical sprays on older cats.

Prior to giving your cat a bath, be certain to brush the hair coat thoroughly to remove any mats and tangles that may be present. In addition, apply some type of protection to prevent corneal burns if shampoo accidentally gets into the eyes. Mineral oil can be used for this purpose; however, a sterile ophthalmic ointment available from your veterinarian or local pet store is preferred. Because many cats are reluctant to be bathed, here are a few tips that may make the job easier:

1. In order to help make your cat feel more secure, consider placing a mat within the tub or sink to provide a surface for your cat to grip onto during the bath.
2. Be sure to fill the tub or sink with lukewarm water prior to introducing your cat to prevent the running water from alarming it.
3. Have containers filled with clean water prepared ahead of time to use for rinsing. If you must turn on the faucet, do so only briefly, then turn it back off.

4. When bathing your cat, keep a firm grip on the top scruff of your pet's neck. Besides offering you greater control, this action (the same that mother cats use to handle their young) alone usually pacifies most cats enough to allow you to complete your task.

5. Following application of the shampoo, be sure to rinse the hair coat thoroughly, concentrating especially on the regions of the armpits, groin, toes, and genitalia, because these are regions commonly missed when rinsing.

6. After the bath is complete, be sure to towel dry your older friend thoroughly.

7. Afterward, apply a commercial ear cleanser (containing a drying agent) to the ears to dry the ear canals.

8. Finally, wait until the coat is completely dry before performing a finishing brush.

Using human nail clippers to trim a cat's nails.

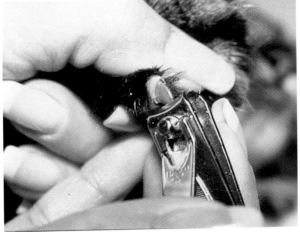

Nail Care

As a general rule, if your older cat has not been previously declawed, its nails should be trimmed every three to four weeks to stimulate healthy growth and to reduce the chances of accidental (or purposeful) scratches being inflicted by your cat.

When trimming nails, use only a brand of nail clipper that is designed for cats. Your pet health care professional can assist you in acquiring such a device. Before trimming a nail, note the line of demarcation between the pink quick (the portion of the nail that contains the blood supply) and the remaining portions of the nail. Using your pair of clippers, snip off the latter portion just in front of the quick. Although ideally you want to avoid drawing blood when you are trimming your cat's nails, don't fret if you do so. Using a clean cloth or towel, simply apply direct pressure to the end of the bleeding nail for three to five minutes. In most cases, this is all that is needed to stop the bleeding, but for stubborn cases, commercially available clotting powder can be applied.

To prevent destruction to household furniture and items, scratching posts should be provided as needed. If your cat has become especially destructive in its later years, disposable nail caps can be glued to your cat's nails to provide a protective barrier against damage from the sharp ends of the nails. Nail cap kits are available at most pet stores or veterinary offices and the caps are relatively easy to apply. The frequency at which you will have to reapply the caps will depend upon the activity level of your cat, and the brand of cap used. All in all, they provide a fantastic (and safe) alternative to surgically removing the claws during the latter years of a cat's life, because declawing can be especially traumatic to the elderly cat.

Ear Care

Routine care for the ears is needed in older cats to prevent moisture, wax, and debris from accumulating within the ear canal and obstructing hearing. Routine examinations of the ears are also useful for detecting infections and other disease conditions early in their development, when they are most easily treated. A good program involves visual examination of the ear canals on a weekly basis, and cleaning and drying with a commercial ear cleanser as needed. Several types of ear cleansers and drying agents are readily available from pet stores, pet supply houses, and veterinary offices. Liquid ear cleansers are preferred over powders, because powders tend to saturate with moisture and become trapped within the ear canal. Most liquid ear cleansers contain both a wax solvent and drying agent (astringent) that clean the ear and dry it at the same time.

If visual examination reveals any signs of irritation, discharges, or

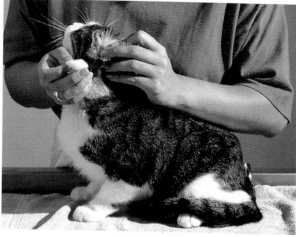

foul odors, your cat's ears should be examined by your veterinarian prior to introducing any liquids or medications in to the ear canals. This is recommended as well for cats that are constantly shaking or tilting their heads. The reason for this is that unhealthy ears may have torn or diseased eardrums, and introducing a cleansing solution into such an ear can spread infection to the deeper portions and structures within the ear.

If your older cat's ears warrant cleaning, begin cleaning by gently pulling the ear flap out and away from the head, exposing and straightening the ear canal. Carefully squeeze a liberal amount of ear cleaning solution into the ear and massage the ear canal for twenty seconds. Next, allow your cat to shake its head, then proceed to the opposite ear and follow the same procedure. Once both ears have been treated, use cotton balls or swabs to remove any wax or debris

A cotton ball can be used to clean the outer portion of the ear canal following use of an ear cleanser.

found on the inside folds of the ear flap and the outer portions of the ear canal. To avoid serious injury to your cat's ear, never enter into the actual ear canal when swabbing.

Dental Care

Keeping your cat's teeth free of tartar and plaque buildup is a preventive health care procedure that will add years to its life. Most cats are afflicted with some degree of tooth and gum disease (periodontal disease) by the time they are three years of age. Not only do plaque-laden teeth and inflamed gums lead to halitosis (foul breath) and eventual tooth loss, but bacteria from these sources can enter the bloodstream and travel to the various organs within the body, including the heart, liver, and kidneys. As a result, regular visits to your veterinarian for professional cleaning and polishing, supplemented by an at-home dental care program, are a must to keep your cat healthy.

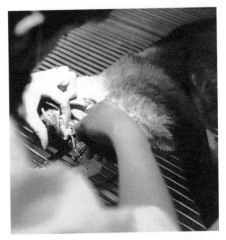

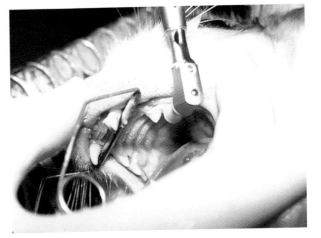

Because a short-acting sedative/anesthetic will be required for professional cleaning, blood tests should be performed on your older cat prior to anesthesia to make certain that there are no underlying conditions that may complicate recovery. Fortunately, recent advancements in veterinary anesthesiology and anesthetic agents have greatly increased the safety of this procedure in elderly felines.

Once anesthetized, an ultrasonic scaler is used to shatter and break up the plaque that has accumulated on your pet's teeth above and below the gum line. After this has been completed, the mouth is rinsed and a polisher is used on the teeth to restore their smooth, shiny surfaces. The entire procedure should take no more than 20 to 30 minutes, after which time your pet will be recovered from the anesthesia.

Professional teeth cleaning such as that described above may be required every four to six months.

However, with diligent dental care provided by you at home on a daily basis, this interval between treatments can be extended to up to one year. Toothpastes and cleansing solutions designed for cats are available from your veterinarian or local pet stores. For best results, use preparations that contain chlorhexidine, an antimicrobial agent that can provide hours of residual protection against bacteria that may attempt to colonize the tooth and gum surfaces. Do not use toothpastes designed for use in humans on your cat; these can cause severe stomach upset in your cat if swallowed. A soft-bristle toothbrush or a rubber fingertip applicator (designed especially for cats and available from your favorite pet store) should be used to gently massage the paste or solution onto the outer, and if possible, inner surfaces of the teeth and gums. At home scaling of dental surfaces using handheld dental scalers should not be performed on cats, because this procedure can be quite painful, and can also create etches and indentations within the tooth surfaces that accelerate tartar buildup.

Neutering Your Older Pet

The term neutering refers to the removal of the ovaries and uterus (ovariohysterectomy, spaying) in the female cat or the testicles (castration) in the male. To reduce the incidence of reproductive disorders and certain types of cancer (including mammary tumors) in later years, it is recommended that all cats be neutered by their eighth birthday. Neutering can also be used to treat select behavioral problems, including aggressiveness and urine spraying, in older cats (see Table 7).

Table 7:
Benefits Associated with Neutering

- Reduced aggressiveness and roaming behavior
    Decreased exposure to feline leukemia (FeLV)/feline immunodeficiency (FIV) disease agents
    Decreased incidence of abscesses
    Reduced stress between cat and owner
- Reduced territorial marking
- Decreased incidence of mammary tumor development
- Elimination of metritis, cystic endometrial hyperplasia, and testicular neoplasia threats
- Feline population control

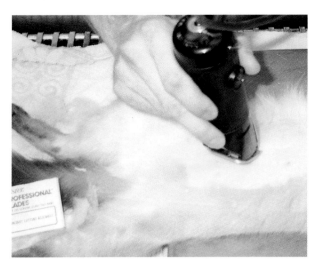

Pre-surgical preparation of a female cat to be neutered.

Sedation and Anesthesia in Older Cats

Sedation and anesthesia are two procedures used to enable veterinarians to perform certain diagnostics and treatments in older cats. *Sedation* refers to the administration of an agent designed to alleviate distress, irritation, excitement, and/or pain in a selected patient. Its primary use in cats is to enable diagnostic procedures such as radiography or endoscopy to be performed without struggle. Sedatives are also effective restraining agents for minor surgical procedures and for therapeutic measures not associated with intense pain. *Anesthesia*, on the other hand, refers to the induction of unconsciousness in a patient using an injectable drug or inhaled gas. Cats in a surgical plane of anesthesia are immune to pain, thereby allowing for more invasive and extensive surgical and therapeutic procedures. In many instances, sedatives are used in conjunction with general anesthetic agents to allow for easier administration of the latter.

With proper preanesthetic blood tests and the use of only the newest, most technologically advanced anesthetic agents, the risks associated with this surgery in an older cat can be greatly reduced. The actual procedure should take no more than 25 minutes to perform. Following postoperative recovery, a physical examination will once again be performed prior to your pet being sent home. Sutures are normally removed seven to ten days following the surgery.

Contrary to popular belief, neutering in itself won't directly cause obesity in cats. Improper feeding practices, lack of exercise, and, in some instances, disease are the causes of obesity in cats, not reproductive status. Furthermore, although it is true that neutering can have a calming effect on nervous or restless cats, activity levels in emotionally stable cats are rarely affected.

There is no doubt that the risks associated with sedation and anesthesia in older cats are much greater than in their younger counterparts. However, with the advent of new, state-of-the-art sedative and anesthetic agents, combined with new diagnostic technology now available to veterinarians, this risk can be reduced significantly. Certainly prior to undergoing any sedation or anesthesia, your cat should be as healthy as possible. A careful physical examination, combined with a complete blood count, biochemistry profile, and urinalysis, should be performed prior to any agent being administered (see Diagnosing Illness in Older Cats and the Interpretation of Laboratory Data following). This will help your veterinarian determine the anesthetic protocol best suited to your pet's condition and reduce the chances of any unexpected surprises. Food should be withheld from cats undergoing anesthesia for a minimum of 12 hours; water for a minimum of 6 hours. Of course, exceptions to these rules may become necessary in cases of emergency. If such an emergency arises, always be sure to inform your veterinarian as to whether or not your cat had eaten or consumed water within these time periods.

Isoflurane is the name of the most technologically advanced form of inhalation anesthesia used in veterinary medicine today. A big advantage of this type of anesthesia over others is that only a very small portion of the agent undergoes metabolism within the body. On the contrary, the majority of this agent is exhaled from the lungs once administration of the gas is ceased. As a result, recovery from isoflurane is usually swift and uneventful. It is certainly the safest agent to use in older cats, especially those with preexisting medical conditions, including heart, liver, and kidney disease. Be sure to request it anytime your pet must undergo anesthesia for dental work or any type of major surgery.

Chapter Four

Diagnosing Illness in Older Cats and Interpreting Laboratory Data

Should your older pet exhibit clinical signs of illness, your veterinarian will follow established diagnostic protocols in an effort to obtain a definitive diagnosis and select the proper treatment. In medical emergencies, nonspecific treatments may be initiated while this diagnostic database is being obtained in order to save precious time.

To begin, your veterinarian will request from you a detailed and thorough history of your pet's problem including but not limited to the time of onset, duration, frequency, and characteristics of the clinical sign(s). The accuracy of this history is essential, because oftentimes it alone can lead to a tentative diagnosis.

After reviewing the history, a physical examination will be performed. Vital physiologic information, including weight, body temperature, pulse, and respiration will usually be obtained first, followed by a systematic, visual and hands-on exam starting at the nose and ending at the tip of the tail. The condition of the heart will be assessed through the use of a stethoscope, and palpation of the chest, abdomen, and limbs will reveal any abnormalities or changes in anatomy and symmetry. Both eyes and ears will be examined using specialized instruments. If clinical signs warrant it, more specialized testing of eye, nervous, and musculoskeletal reflexes and functions may be performed during the physical exam as well.

If the history and physical examination fail to uncover the exact cause of your cat's clinical signs, further diagnostic testing will be needed. Oftentimes, due to financial considerations, pet owners may opt to forgo any further diagnostics and treat the clinical signs instead of identifying and treating the underlying disease. Although a small percentage of pets may respond to such an approach, most will not. As a result, be prepared to

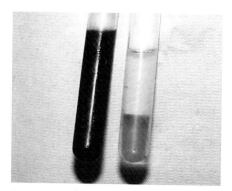

trust and follow your veterinarian when it comes to diagnostic protocols and recommendations.

Complete blood counts (CBC) and serum biochemical profiles performed on samples of your pet's blood provide valuable insights into the inner workings of the organ systems of the body (see Tables 8–10). For instance, a CBC can be useful in diagnosing anemia, inflammatory and infectious diseases, and blood-clotting disorders. Serum biochemistry profiles can identify increases or decreases in organ-specific enzymes, metabolic by-products, minerals, and electrolytes within the blood that may occur secondary to disease. Because most of these changes can be correlated with specific diseases, this analysis is invaluable toward the establishment of a conclusive diagnosis.

Whenever a cat is presented for an illness, your veterinarian will want to perform blood tests for FeLV and FIV if such testing has not been done within the past six to eight months. Because of the widespread prevalence and importance of these two diseases, even cats that have

been previously vaccinated against FeLV and those that are kept exclusively indoors should be tested if clinical signs lead to suspicions of either disease. Establishing a cat's FeLV/FIV status before extensive diagnostics and treatments are performed will save time and money, and help your veterinarian choose the best course of action to take toward managing or curing your cat's immediate illness.

In addition to a generalized analysis of your cat's blood, laboratory analysis of the urine also provides valuable clues when attempting to pin down the cause of an illness. Kidney disease, liver disease, diabetes mellitus, bleeding disorders, FUS, and poisonings are just some of the conditions that can be reflected in a urinalysis. Urine samples submitted for testing should be obtained at your veterinarian's office to ensure freshness and accuracy of the results (see Table 11, page 46).

Microscopic examination of your pet's stool is almost always performed in a general diagnostic package, especially if your pet is exhibiting signs of gastrointestinal illness. Not only will such a test help reveal internal parasites that may be causing the illness, but the nature and content of the feces may be diagnostic for certain poisonings and dietary indiscretions. To ensure accurate results, your veterinarian will require the freshest sample possible, and if necessary can obtain one in-house.

Table 8: Components of a Complete Blood Count (CBC)

Hematocrit (Hct)
Hematocrit, or packed cell volume, is the ratio of red blood cells to total blood volume. Decreases in the hematocrit are caused by anemia, which can have several underlying sources, including FeLV. Increases are seen with dehydration, myeloproliferative disorders, lung disease, and cardiomyopathy.

Red blood cell (RBC) count
Decreases in the red blood cell count are indicative of anemia, which can have several underlying causes. Increases in red blood cell numbers can be caused by dehydration, lung disease, myeloproliferative disorders, and cardiomyopathy.

Hemoglobin (Hb) concentration
Hemoglobin is the molecule found in red blood cells that is responsible for transport of oxygen molecules. Increases and decreases in Hb concentration usually follow those of Hct and RBC count.

Mean corpuscular volume (MCV)
MCV is the ratio of the Hct to the RBC count. Increases in MCV are caused by vitamin deficiencies, decreases are caused by iron deficiencies.

Mean corpuscular hemoglobin concentration (MCHC)
MCHC is the ratio of Hb concentration to the hematocrit. As with MCV, decreases in MCHC result from iron deficiencies and from an increase in reticulocyte counts. Increases in MCHC occur secondary to red blood cell destruction within the body.

Reticulocyte count
Reticulocytes are immature red blood cells that appear in response to anemia. A high reticulocyte count in the presence of anemia indicates that the body is attempting to replace the lost red blood cells. In contrast, a low reticulocyte count in the presence of anemia indicates that the body is unable, for whatever reason, to respond to the anemic state.

Blood smears and blood cell morphology
These smears, when stained and evaluated under the microscope, reveal size and shape abnormalities of red blood cells, white blood cell numbers and types, and platelet counts. Red blood cell abnormalities can be caused by inflammation, myeloproliferative disorders, and nutritional deficiencies.

White blood cell count
The total white blood cell count in a blood sample can help determine whether or not inflammation or infection is occurring within an individual. Increases in white blood cell numbers are usually seen with inflammation, infection, or neoplasia. Decreases in white blood cell numbers may occur with long-term, overwhelming infections, certain viral diseases such as feline panleukopenia, and poisoning.

White blood cell differentiation and percentages
Along with a total white blood cell count, a CBC will usually break down into percentages of total count the five different types of white blood cells that exist. Neutrophils should make up the greatest percentage of white blood cells in a sample, followed by lymphocytes, monocytes, eosinophils, and basophils. Increases in neutrophil numbers are seen with stress, excitement, inflammation, infections with bacteria, fungi, or viruses, parasitic infestations, tissue damage, neoplasia, and autoimmune disease. Decreases may be indicative of a severe bacterial infection, certain viral infections, toxins, and bone marrow disorders. Lymphocyte percentages can increase with lymphosarcoma, allergies, autoimmune disease, Addison's disease, and myeloproliferative disorders, or following routine vaccinations. Declines in lymphocyte counts can occur secondary to endocrine diseases, such as Cushing's disease, chemotherapy for neoplasia, chylothorax, or any long-standing, stressful disease or disorder. Monocyte levels are increased with chronic infections, heartworms, fungal diseases, autoimmune disease, trauma, stress, and neoplasia. Decreases in monocyte numbers are not clinically significant. Elevations in eosinophil numbers in older cats are usually seen with parasitic infestations, allergies, and tumors, whereas decreases occur secondarily to stress and early inflammation or infection. Finally, basophils are rarely found in the bloodstream and when they are, can be indicative of heartworm disease, allergic skin disease, and/or neoplasia.

Platelet count
Platelets serve a vital role in the body's blood-clotting mechanism. Decreases in platelet numbers, or interference with their function can lead to uncontrolled hemorrhage. Decreases in the number of platelets in any given blood sample result from autoimmune disease, excessive consumption due to internal bleeding or clotting, chemotherapy, and bone marrow disorders, including myeloproliferative disorders.

Table 9: Components of a Biochemical Profile and Their Interpretation

Blood urea nitrogen (BUN)
Blood urea nitrogen is a by-product of protein metabolism within the body. Increases in BUN can be caused by dehydration, kidney disease, cardiovascular disease, and shock. Decreases in BUN can be seen in liver disease.

Serum creatinine
Creatinine is a compound made from amino acids. The amount of creatinine in the blood is closely regulated by the kidneys. As a result, abnormal elevations of this substance in the blood is indicative of kidney disease.

Glucose
Glucose is the sugar that is the primary source of energy within the body. Marked increases in the glucose content of the blood can occur with diabetes mellitus, Cushing's disease, stress, drug therapy, convulsions, and excitement, and within hours after a meal. Decreases in glucose levels can be seen with liver disease, advanced seizure activity, Addison's disease, gastrointestinal disease, parasitism, starvation, and neoplasia.

Sodium
This chemical element is important to the fluid balance within the body. Increases in sodium are caused by dehydration and high fever. Decreases are seen in Addison's disease, vomiting, diarrhea, starvation, kidney disease, diabetes mellitus, and bladder disease.

Potassium
Potassium is another chemical element found within the body. Increases in potassium levels are seen with Addison's disease, tissue damage, dehydration, and oversupplementation. Diminished amounts of potassium in the blood occur secondarily to vomiting, diarrhea, stress, drug therapy (insulin, diuretics), malnutrition, and kidney disease.

Chloride
Chloride is a salt within the body that is also important to the water and pH balance within the body. Increases can be caused by diarrhea, kidney disease, diabetes mellitus, and shock. Decreases in chloride levels occur secondarily to vomiting, diarrhea, and malnutrition.

Calcium

The most abundant mineral within the body, calcium is important for muscle function, heart function, blood clotting, nerve conduction, and integrity of the teeth and bones. Tumors, hyperparathyroidism, Addison's disease, bone infections, and kidney failure can all cause increases in blood calcium levels. Decreases in calcium levels are seen with pancreatitis and low blood protein levels.

Phosphorus

This chemical element helps run important metabolic processes throughout the body. It also contributes to the structural integrity of bone. Elevations are seen with bone tumors, kidney disease, and hypoparathyroidism. Decreases are caused by hyperparathyroidism, tumors, and poor nutrition.

Total serum protein

Total serum protein levels refer to levels of albumin, which is a transport protein within the blood, and globulin proteins, which are important for transporting substances in the blood and for immunity. Increases in total protein levels result from dehydration and immune responses to infection. Decreases in serum protein are seen with immunodeficiency disease, gastrointestinal disease, parasitism, pancreatic disease, liver disease, kidney disease, blood loss, Addison's disease, and severe skin disease.

Creatinine phosphokinase (CPK)

Not to be confused with serum creatinine, CPK is an enzyme located primarily in muscle and brain tissue. Elevations in this enzyme occur with muscle disease and trauma.

Lactic dehydrogenase (LDH)

LDH is an enzyme found in the cell membranes of most tissues, especially the kidneys, muscle, and liver. Serum elevations are seen with muscle disease, liver disease, heart disease, red blood cell destruction, and tissue necrosis.

Asparate aminotransferase (AST, SGOT)

This enzyme is found in tissues throughout the body, including the heart, liver, muscle, and blood. Increases in AST are caused by liver, heart, and muscle disease.

Alanine aminotransferase (ALT, SGPT)

ALT is a liver-specific enzyme. As a result, elevations in this enzyme are indicative of liver disease, specifically damage to the liver tissue itself.

Alkaline phosphatase (ALP, SAP)

Alkaline phosphatase is an enzyme found on cell membranes throughout the body. Elevations of this substance are most commonly seen with liver disease, Cushing's disease, steroid drug therapy, hyperparathyroidism, and neoplasia.

Bilirubin

Bilirubin is a pigment found in blood and in bile. It is produced by the liver, originating from the breakdown of the oxygen-carrying molecules found in red blood cells (hemoglobin) and muscle tissue (myoglobin). Increases are seen in liver disease, red blood cell destruction, muscle disease, and trauma.

Bile acids

These compounds are derived from cholesterol and produced in the liver. They are responsible for the absorption of fat from the small intestine. Abnormalities in the amount of bile acids detected in the blood stream is indicative of liver disease.

Cholesterol

Cholesterol is a steroid compound produced primarily by the liver that is vital to normal cellular structure and function. Increases occur with kidney disease, liver disease, Cushing's disease, gastrointestinal disease, diabetes mellitus, and pancreatitis. Decreases in normal levels usually occur because of improper fat digestion.

Gamma glutamyltransferase (GGT)

GGT is found in the liver, kidney, and pancreas. Elevations in this enzyme are usually attributable to liver disease, steroid drug therapy, or treatment with anticonvulsant medications.

Amylase

Amylase is an enzyme produced in the pancreas and is also found in the liver and intestinal lining. It functions in the normal digestion of nutrients. Elevations are seen with pancreatic disease, kidney failure, Cushing's disease, liver disease, and gastrointestinal disease.

Lipase

Lipase is an enzyme produced by the pancreas and by the lining of the stomach. Increases in serum levels can be caused by pancreatic disease, kidney failure, Cushing's disease, liver disease, and gastrointestinal disease.

Table 10: Correlation of Clinical Disease with Biochemical Changes

Disease Condition	Look for Changes in:
Kidney disease	BUN Serum creatinine Sodium Potassium Phosphorus Calcium
Liver disease	ALT AST ALP GGT Bilirubin Bile acids Glucose Cholesterol
Adrenal gland disease	ALP ALT AST Glucose Cholesterol Sodium Potassium Phosphorus Calcium
Muscle disease	CPK AST LDH Bilirubin
Pancreatic disease	Amylase Lipase
Bone disease	Calcium Phosphorus

Table 11: The Urinalysis and Its Interpretation

Volume
In older cats, the volume of urine produced is important information if kidney disease is suspected. In cats suffering from actual kidney failure, urine volume is an important parameter in the determination of a prognosis.

Color and appearance
Normal urine is yellow to amber in color, the intensity of which depends upon its water content. Cats that are dehydrated will have dark yellow urine as the body attempts to conserve water. In contrast, urine that is so light in color that it resembles water may simply indicate overhydration, or more seriously, it could indicate that the kidneys are unable to concentrate the urine with filtered wastes. Urine that is red in appearance contains blood, whereas orange-colored or brown urine may also indicate the presence of blood, as well as hemoglobin or myoglobin, the latter of which shows up as the result of muscle trauma. Greenish-tinged urine is seen with increased amounts of bilirubin or with certain bacterial infections. Finally, normal urine is clear and transparent to the naked eye. Cloudy urine can be seen with increased amounts of blood cells, bacteria, fungi, mucus, spermatozoa, and crystals.

Specific gravity
Specific gravity measures the amount and weight of substances found in the urine. As the kidneys concentrate the urine with waste material, specific gravity should increase. In addition, dehydration will normally cause an increase in this parameter. Low specific gravity, indicating dilute urine, in itself doesn't necessarily mean disease is present; however, repeated readings of a low specific gravity in combination with dehydration usually means kidney disease is present. In addition, other disease conditions that can cause a low urine specific gravity include liver disease, Cushing's disease, diabetes mellitus, and pyometra.

pH
The pH of a cat's urine is normally acidic in nature, except for a brief period of time after the consumption of a meal. Alkaline urine with a pH above 7.5 that is not associated with a meal is usually indicative of a urinary tract infection or bacterial contamination of the urine sample. It is important to note, however, that bacterial infections can exist in an acidic pH as well.

Protein
Under normal conditions, the urine of a cat should contain only trace amounts of protein. Any measurable increases can occur due to kidney disease, hemoglobin or myoglobin in the urine, inflammatory debris, and blood cells.

Glucose
Glucose should not be measurable in the urine of healthy cats. Glucose in the urine is most often caused by diabetes mellitus. Other etiologies can include pancreatitis, Cushing's disease, kidney failure, stress and excitement, and certain tumors.

Ketones
Ketones are formed when abnormalities in fat and energy metabolism occur; as a result, they should not be found in the urine of normal cats. Persistent fever, starvation, and diabetes mellitus can all lead to the appearance of ketones in the urine.

Occult blood
The presence of occult blood in the urine indicates the presence of red blood cells, hemoglobin, or myoglobin.

White blood cells
Although the results of this test may be less than reliable, the presence of white blood cells in the urine is indicative of a urinary tract infection.

Bilirubin
Bilirubin may be present in trace amounts in the urine of healthy cats. However, elevated amounts indicate red blood cell destruction within the body or liver disease.

Urine sediment
Microscopic analysis of the sediment formed by centrifuging a urine sample is useful in identifying white blood cells, red blood cells, bacteria, urinary crystals, casts, and epithelial cells. Urinary crystals often form as a result of FUS (see Feline Urologic Syndrome, page 86). Casts are cylindrical accumulations of cells and/or debris that occur secondary to kidney disease. Finally, abnormal amounts of epithelial cells from the kidneys or bladder are indicative of inflammation, infection, or neoplasia affecting these organs

Cytology is a newer diagnostic tool being utilized more and more by veterinarians. *Cytology* refers to the microscopic examination of fluids, discharges, lesions, or masses for cells and debris that may be characteristic of specific illnesses and conditions. The substance to be observed cytologically is obtained via a needle and syringe or swab and applied to a microscope slide for special staining and preparation. Because of the importance and significance of this valuable diagnostic tool, veterinarians today are receiving extensive training in this field in order to provide pet owners with this state-of-the-art diagnostic technology.

One step up from cytology, biopsies are actual tissue samples from organs and structures within the body removed by surgical or endoscopic methods. Once removed, these samples are fixed in formalin, then prepared in the laboratory for microscopic viewing. Biopsies are

Contrast radiograph of the intestines of a cat.

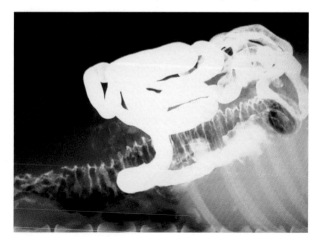

especially useful in identifying and staging neoplasia that may affect senior felines.

Radiographs, often incorrectly referred to as X-rays, are pictorial representations of bones and internal organs within the body. They are created by passing X-ray radiation through a specific portion of the body that has been placed over special radiographic film. A portion of the X-rays will be fully or partially absorbed by the body structures, whereas others are allowed to pass through unimpeded. This results in an outline image of the structure in question created on the film, providing an anatomical picture that can be used for diagnostic purposes. Older cats, especially those suffering from injury or illness, can be challenging to radiograph, because they will rarely remain motionless while a radiograph is being taken. As a result, sedation or anesthesia is often needed to provide the restraint needed for quality radiographs.

In some instances, plain radiographs by themselves may not be able to provide enough anatomic detail to uncover answers to your pet's problem. In these instances, special contrast materials such as barium or radiographic iodine may be administered orally or by enema, or may be injected directly into a lesion. X rays are unable to penetrate these materials; as a result, they appear white on a radiograph, providing an excellent outline of the organ or lesion in question.

Another strategy that is becoming popular as an adjunct to radiographs is endoscopy. *Endoscopy* is performed using a special tool called an endoscope. This instrument consists of a long, narrow, flexible tube containing fiber optics and special channels that are attached to a light source and a magnifier. With an endoscope, a veterinarian can examine most hollow organs, as well as body cavities, with minimal invasiveness and trauma. Endoscopes are commonly used to assess the overall health of an organ or cavity, to obtain biopsy samples, and to retrieve foreign objects from the respiratory and digestive tracts. In some cases, it can provide an effective alternative to surgical intervention.

Ultrasonography is a diagnostic method that utilizes sound waves to outline internal organs and structures. Upon scanning a portion of the body, ultrasonic sound waves produce an image on a special screen that can be interpreted by a trained veterinarian. Ultrasonography is especially useful in identifying tumors within the body, as well as heart abnormalities. It is an excellent diagnostic tool, because it is simple, safe, and noninvasive.

Finally, *exploratory surgery* can become useful in diagnostics when all other tests and procedures have failed to reveal an answer to a pet's illness. Although there certainly are inherent risks in exploratory surgery they must be weighed against the risks of failing to definitively diag-

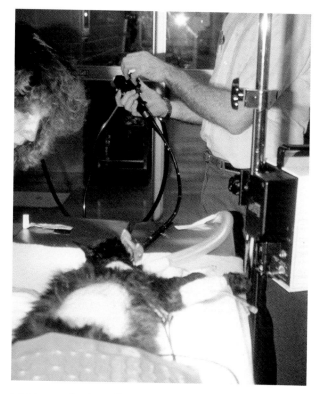

Endoscopy is a useful tool in diagnosing digestive system disorders in older cats.

nose an elusive disease condition. By performing a physical examination, CBC, biochemistry profile, and urinalysis prior to the surgery, veterinarians are able to assess a cat's inherent surgical risk and help reduce these risks to a minimum.

Numerous other specialized tests can also be employed in the event of an elusive diagnosis. Table 12 lists additional diagnostic tests that may be ordered if your cat is suffering from a less-than-obvious illness. Because each pet's condition should be considered unique, the protocol and tests used by a veterinarian may or may not include those presented here.

Table 12: Specialized Diagnostic Tests Utilized in Veterinary Medicine

Diagnostic Test	Target System/Group Tests for:
Cardiovascular and pulmonary system	
Heartworm antigen test	Feline heartworm disease
Electrocardiogram (ECG)	Abnormal electrical activity within the heart
Bleeding profile	Blood-clotting disorders
Blood gas profile	pH imbalances within the body
Angiogram	Circulation disturbances
Bone marrow analysis	Abnormalities in the production of blood cells; myeloproliferative disorders
Urinary and reproductive systems	
Endogenous creatinine clearance test	Abnormalities in kidney filtration rates
Vaginal/urethral flush and cytology	Infections, tumors
Musculoskeletal system	
Electromyogram (EMG)	Abnormal muscle activity
Joint cytology/cultures	Arthritis
Nervous system	
Electroencephalogram (EEG)	Abnormal electrical activity within the brain
Neurologic examination	Abnormalities in neurologic reflex activity
Cerebrospinal fluid analysis/culture	Infectious diseases; inflammation
Myelogram	Degenerative disk disease; spinal cord disorders
Magnetic resonance imaging (MRI)	Brain or spinal cord lesions
Computed tomography (CT scan)	Brain or spinal cord lesions

Endocrine system

Thyroid hormone profile (T3,T4, TSH stimulation)	Hyperthyroidism
ACTH stimulation test/ Plasma ACTH concentrations	Cushing's disease, Addison's disease
Insulin/glucose ratio	Diabetes mellitus

Gastrointestinal system

Fecal trypsin test	Poor fat digestion
Food allergy trial	Food allergies
BT-PABA test	Pancreatic disease
Xylose absorption test	Intestinal disease
Sudan/iodine staining of feces	Pancreatic disease

Skin and hair coat

Skin scrape	Mange mites
Dermatophyte test medium (DTM)	Ringworm
Allergy testing	Specific skin allergies
Autoimmune profile	Autoimmune skin diseases

Immune system

Antinuclear antibody (ANA) test	Autoimmune disease
Lupus erythematosus (LE) test	Autoimmune disease
Rheumatoid factor	Autoimmune disease
Bone marrow analysis	Abnormalities in the production of immune cells; myeloproliferative disorders

Eyes

Schirmer tear test	Inadequate tear film production
Tonometry	Glaucoma
Electroretinogram (ERG)	Abnormalities in retinal function
Corneal staining	Ulcers on the cornea

Infectious diseases

Serum antigen tests	Specific disease agents (such as FeLV)
Antibody titers	Antibodies to specific disease agents (FIV)
Culture/sensitivity	Specific organisms/sensitivity to antimicrobial drugs

Chapter Five

Select Diseases and Disorders Affecting the Body Systems of Older Cats

In focusing attention on select illnesses that are often seen in older cats, it is important to remember that these conditions only touch the surface of the entire range of geriatric diseases and disorders. A proper diagnostic protocol performed by a qualified veterinarian is still essential to ensure proper identification of any illness.

Older cats that are ill will often have oily, rough hair coats.

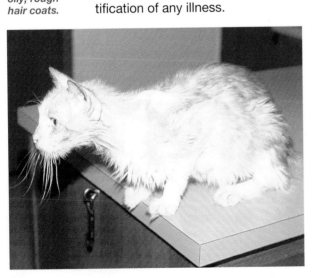

Viral Diseases

Viruses can cause a number of serious diseases in older cats. These unique entities consist of genetic material wrapped in a protein coating. After infecting a cell, viruses seize control of the cell's internal functions for the sole purpose of replicating and thereby propagating the infection to other cells throughout the body. Damage to and death of the host cell can occur not only from the activity of the virus within the cell, but also from the immune response mounted by the body against the invader. In addition, some viruses will enter a dormant stage within the body whereby they "hide" from the host's immune system and cause little, if any, clinical signs. This stage can sometimes last for years at a time before the virus becomes active again, often secondary to stress or other disease conditions.

What makes viral infections so challenging is that there are relatively few medications that are effective against them. At best, those antiviral agents that are available exhibit very generalized activity against the infectious agents, and are often cost prohibitive for many pet owners. For these reasons and others, the body's own immune system should be considered the primary line of defense against viruses. Routine vaccinations combined with excellent nutrition and controlled stress are the most effective means of keeping the immune system primed and in top shape should it be called into action against a viral infection. In addition, limiting exposure to known sources of the viral particles is also a definitive way of protecting a pet against these disease agents.

Feline Leukemia Virus (FeLV)

Feline leukemia virus (FeLV) has become one of the most important diseases affecting the feline population of this country. Caused by an oncogenic (tumor-producing) retrovirus, FeLV can produce devastating disease in affected cats. The virus can itself incorporate into the genetic material of the cells it infects, providing instant reproduction whenever the infected cell reproduces. This characteristic is but one of many that make this disease especially challenging to its host.

FeLV is spread by close contact between cats, being present in

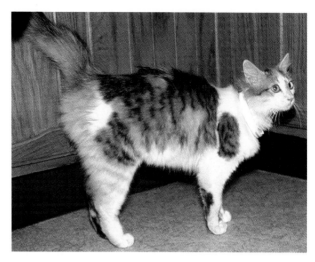

almost all types of body fluids, including saliva, urine, feces, blood, and respiratory secretions. Saliva seems to be an effective carrier of the virus, causing social grooming, bite wounds, and shared food bowls to be important methods of transmission. Because cats can carry the FeLV for extended periods of time without exhibiting clinical signs, they may become silent transmitters of the infection to other felines.

In certain regions of the country, the incidence of FeLV in cat-owning households is as high as 30 percent! Although the incidence of FeLV is much less in older cats than it is in their younger counterparts, they are still very susceptible to infection, especially as the efficiency of the immune system declines with advancing age. Many types of drug therapy commonly used in older pets can also decrease the body's ability to resist infection if exposure indeed occurs.

Feline leukemia is the number one infectious disease of cats today.

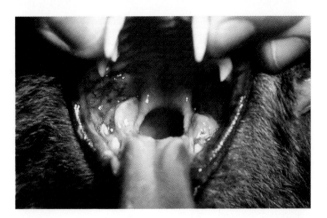

Swollen tonsils associated with FeLV-induced lymphosarcoma.

Upon gaining entrance into the body via the mouth or nose, FeLV infects lymphatic tissue, or more specifically, lymphocytes located in these regions. From here, the virus spreads to the bone marrow and other lymphatic tissue throughout the body, where massive replication takes place. Suppression of bone marrow activity often occurs as a result of the viral infection, predisposing the body to the development of cancer, anemia, or a wide variety of secondary diseases associated with immunosuppression. In addition, while in the bone marrow, the virus will infect other white blood cells and platelets, and gain entrance into the bloodstream, causing a viremia and spreading to various tissues throughout the body. Once the virus gains access to these distant tissues, the chances of the viral infection being eliminated by the cat's own immune system are all but gone.

Due to the multisystem involvement of this disease and the character of the virus, the clinical signs associated with FeLV infection can be quite varied (see Table 13). Some infected cats exhibit no clinical signs whatsoever, with the virus remaining latent within the bone marrow. However, these latent infections may suddenly become active in response to stress or therapy with select drugs. With active infections, clinical signs seen will usually be related to the secondary diseases caused by the virus's immunosuppressive nature. Gingivitis and severe periodontal disease, respiratory infections, skin infections, ear infections, abscesses, swollen lymph nodes, and recurring bladder infections are all commonly seen in cats suffering from FeLV. Vomiting and diarrhea as well as dehydration may appear as the disease exerts its effects on the stomach, intestines, and kidneys. Symptoms associated with anemia (such as weakness, loss of appetite, and pale mucous membranes) are also quite prevalent in FeLV-infected cats; in fact, FeLV is the most common cause of anemia in cats. Finally, secondary infections with FIP, FIV, and toxoplasmosis and associated symptoms have been documented in cats infected with FeLV, as have cases of secondary kidney disease.

A number of specific laboratory tests can be used to diagnose feline leukemia in cats. One such test is the enzyme-linked immunosorbent assay (ELISA). This procedure can be used to detect FeLV antigen in a cat's blood, saliva, or tears. ELISA is useful in detecting early infections with the virus, even before bone

Table 13:
FeLV-Associated
Diseases and Syndromes

- Lymphosarcoma
- Myeloproliferative/bone marrow disorders
- Anemia
- White blood cell suppression
- Glomerulonephritis and kidney failure
- FIV
- FIP
- Toxoplasmosis
- Periodontal disease
- Recurring abscesses
- Poor wound healing
- Colitis
- Recurring respiratory infections
- Recurring urinary infections
- Ear infections

marrow infection has taken place. Most veterinarians are equipped to perform an ELISA test for FeLV right in their clinic or hospital. A second type of test, called an immunofluorescence assay (IFA), can also detect the presence of FeLV antigen in a blood sample, yet it is more specific for detecting later stages of infection when the virus has infected the bone marrow and white blood cells. Because this test is much more involved than the ELISA test, blood samples must be sent out to specialized laboratories for this test to be performed.

A positive ELISA test result means that an infection has taken place, yet it doesn't mean that the patient is permanently infected with the virus. For this reason, a second ELISA test should always be performed 12 weeks after the first test if the former comes back positive. If the second test comes back negative, this means that the cat's immune system has successfully eliminated the virus. However, if it reads positive like the first test, then most likely the cat is permanently infected with the virus. At this stage, an IFA test is usually performed to verify whether or not this is indeed true. If the IFA test returns negative even after the second ELISA test, then this usually means that the cat is still carrying the FeLV virus, yet the infection has become dormant. Cats that are ELISA positive and IFA negative are usually noncontagious to other cats and have a decreased susceptibility to the ill effects and diseases caused by FeLV. On the other hand, if the IFA test returns positive, then it is safe to assume that the cat will be a carrier of the virus for the remainder of its life and can spread the disease to other cats. Cats that are both ELISA positive and IFA positive are at greatest risk of developing FeLV-associated illnesses and diseases (see Table 14).

Because feline leukemia is caused by a viral organism, there is no specific treatment available to combat this disease. Treatment is geared toward the FeLV-associated diseases as they arise, and many times is merely supportive in nature.

Table 14: Interpretation of FeLV Test Results

ELISA positive/IFA negative

The FeLV virus is in blood, yet has not reached the bone marrow. These cats are rarely contagious to other cats and have a low susceptibility to the development of FeLV-related disease.

ELISA positive/IFA positive

The FeLV virus has reached the bone marrow and infected cells therein. These cats usually remain contagious carriers of the disease for life and are very prone to the development of FeLV-related disease.

ELISA negative/IFA positive

Both tests should be repeated to ensure accurate results. If the follow-up test results are the same, then it can be assumed that the cat is permanently infected with the FeLV virus, yet may not be contagious to other cats. However, it is still highly susceptible to FeLV-related disease.

The goals of any treatment regimen for cats suffering ill effects from feline leukemia include the alleviation of clinical signs and maintaining an acceptable quality of life. Blood transfusions, intravenous fluids, and antibiotics can all be employed for this purpose, depending upon the clinical signs that are present and any internal manifestations that may arise. For lymphosarcoma and other tumors that may result from FeLV infection, chemotherapy is indicated in an effort to achieve remission. Special drugs designed to stimulate the immune system have been used with mixed results in an attempt to help the infected cat's own body fight off the disease. The drug interferon has also been employed to help abate clinical symptoms, yet has not proven effective at clearing an infection. Unfortunately, for those cats with bone marrow infections, over 50 percent will succumb to the disease within six months after the onset of clinical signs regardless of supportive therapy; over 80 percent will die within 48 months, often due to secondary kidney failure brought about by the disease.

Due to the serious nature of feline leukemia and lack of effective treatment, all cats should be vaccinated against this deadly disease agent. An ELISA test should be performed prior to vaccination in order to confirm an FeLV-negative health status, because vaccinating an FeLV-positive cat serves no purpose and may create a false sense of security. Also, cats that are unknowingly harboring the FeLV virus certainly pose a threat to other felines. For this reason, all new cats and kittens that are brought into a household should be tested by both the ELISA and IFA methods to be certain that they pose no health threat to an existing cat in the household, especially an older one.

If an FeLV-negative cat or kitten is to be brought in to a household containing an FeLV-positive cat, it should be completely vaccinated (including a complete booster series) prior to coming in contact with the infected cat. Also, even though a new cat may be vaccinated for FeLV, it still should be fed from its own food and water bowls.

When discussing feline leukemia, the question of transmissibility to human beings arises quite often. To date, there is no known evidence to show that FeLV can be transmitted to humans from infected cats. However, much still remains unknown concerning retroviruses and their activity. As a result, many researchers do encourage restricting human exposure to IFA-positive cats. This is especially true for young children, the elderly, and immunocompromised individuals (i.e., those receiving chemotherapy or recovering from a debilitating disease). In addition, after handling a cat infected with the feline leukemia virus, good hygiene is always recommended.

Feline Immunodeficiency Virus (FIV)

In 1987, researchers discovered a new disease-causing virus in cats—the feline immunodeficiency virus (FIV)—that adversely affects the immune system of the host it infects. This virus belongs to a special class of retroviruses called *lentiviruses* (including the virus that causes acquired immunodeficiency

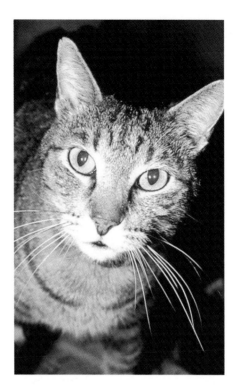

Stray tomcats within a neighborhood are important carriers of FIV.

syndrome [AIDS] in humans). Lentiviruses are well known for their ability to compromise a host's immune system, leaving the body open to attack from foreign organisms and more susceptible to malignancies. Upon discovery, it was found that FIV actually is quite widespread among the cat population throughout the world. The prevalence of this disease among cats is as low as 1 percent in certain locations to as high as 35 percent or more in select neighborhoods. The virus causes clinical disease syndromes similar to those caused by the feline leukemia virus, namely anemia, low white blood cell counts, and chronic recurring

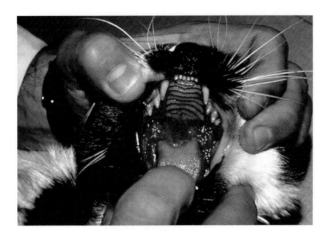

these nodes. The virus then spreads to lymph nodes throughout the body, oftentimes causing noticeable enlargements in these nodes at various points on the body. Over weeks to years, signs of pronounced immunodeficiency begin to occur, including a suppression of the body's red and white cell counts, and the appearance of secondary infections by otherwise innocuous organisms. Stomatitis, gingivitis, emaciation, general unthriftiness, periodontal disease, low-grade fever, weakness (related to anemia), and repeated infections involving the skin, urinary tract, and respiratory system can all be seen with a maturing FIV infection. Less commonly, seizures and other neurologic signs may be present in select cases. Lastly, all symptoms associated with FIV may become cyclical in nature; that is, they may appear for a short period of time and then regress, only to resurface at a later date.

infections. However, unlike the feline leukemia virus, FIV is not known to actively stimulate the formation of tumors.

Like the feline leukemia virus, FIV has the ability to insert its genetic material into that of its host's cells, setting the stage for virus replication each time the host cell undergoes division. The virus may then remain dormant for years before actually causing immunosuppression and clinical disease. As a result, many cats receive exposure to the disease through contact with inapparent (clinically healthy) carriers.

The primary mode through which this exposure occurs is through deep bite wounds received during an aggressive encounter with a carrier cat. Free-roaming, nonneutered male cats are the most common carriers of the disease, due to their fighting tendencies. Once the virus is implanted deep within the tissues, it spreads to the regional lymph nodes and begins replicating within the lymphocytes residing in

Diagnosis of an FIV infection is based upon a history of potential exposure, clinical signs, and a special diagnostic test that can be performed on a sample of blood right in a veterinary office. This test is designed to detect antibodies to the FIV virus that may be circulating in the cat's blood. Because of the serious nature of this disease, positive results from this test should be substantiated by a second test performed by a regional veterinary diagnostic lab. In addition, because it may take 8 to 12 weeks following exposure to the virus before antibodies will become detectable within the blood, those cats that are suspected of having FIV and yet exhibit a negative antibody test should be retested 6 to 8 weeks after the first test was performed.

Cats suffering from clinical signs and disease brought about by an FIV infection can be treated with antibiotics, antifungal medications, intravenous fluids, and/or blood transfusions as warranted by their condition. Furthermore, high-calorie diets can be used to help counteract the catabolic (breaking down) effects of this disease. Also, the experimental drug AZT has been used with mixed results to help lengthen the life of cats showing signs of immunodeficiency related to the feline immunodeficiency virus. However, because AZT is expensive and can have significant side effects when used in felines, use in FIV cats is restricted.

Because there is no specific treatment for FIV in cats, preventive measures should be taken to reduce your cat's risk of exposure to this deadly disease. The prevention of night roaming, when most cat-to-cat fighting occurs, and close monitoring of outdoor activity will help minimize social interactions that may take place between a healthy cat and an FIV carrier.

To date, there is no evidence that the feline immunodeficiency virus poses a health threat to human beings. However, it is recommended that those persons with a potential immune compromise (cancer patients receiving chemotherapy; organ transplant recipients) or those young children whose immune systems may not be working at their peak capacities should be kept apart from cats known to be infected with FIV.

Feline Upper Respiratory Disease (FURD)

Infections involving the nasal passages and upper airways are all classified under the heading of feline upper respiratory disease (FURD). FURD can appear in those elderly cats stressed by disease or poorly functioning immune systems, as well as those not kept current on their vaccinations. At least six infectious disease agents, possibly more, can contribute to the development of upper respiratory disease in cats. Of these, the two main agents responsible for the most severe clinical disease include the feline herpesvirus and the feline calicivirus. FURD caused by the feline herpesvirus is known as *feline rhinotracheitis*, characterized by marked inflammation within the nose and trachea. This is a highly contagious disease spread through infective droplets sneezed from the airways of infected cats that gain access into the body via the mouth, nose, and eyes. Contact with infected food and water bowls, litter boxes, and the contaminated clothing and hands of an owner is another common mode of transmission of this virus from cat to cat.

The *feline calicivirus* causes a disease syndrome in cats similar to the common cold in humans. It too is transmitted through infective respiratory droplets. In addition, the virus can contaminate the urine and feces of infected cats, thereby spreading in this manner. Interestingly enough, both the herpesvirus and calicivirus can remain within a host cat for long periods of time even after clinical signs of disease have abated. In many instances, these "carrier" cats may shed the viruses for months and serve as a source of infection for other felines. In addition to these two viruses, a nonviral organism called *Chlamydia psittaci* can also play a prominent role in the development of FURD in certain regions of the country. This is the same organism that can cause respiratory disease in psittacine birds and in humans. Cats afflicted with infectious upper respiratory disease may be harboring more than one disease agent at the same time.

Clinical signs associated with infection by any one of these upper respiratory agents can include sneezing, coughing, depression, decreased appetite, red eyes with discharge, and nasal discharges. This latter discharge usually starts off clear in nature and may become mucoid and crusty if secondary bacterial infection occurs. Ulcerations affecting the tongue and gums may become apparent as well, leading to halitosis and excessive salivation. Allowed to progress unchecked, FURD can spread to the lower parts of the respiratory system and, along with secondary bacterial infections, cause permanent damage and scarring.

Diagnosis of upper respiratory disease is achieved by evaluating the history of exposure, clinical signs, and physical examination findings. In addition, cells and fluids collected from the membranes surrounding the eyes, nose, and throat can be used in an attempt to isolate and identify the organisms involved. Because a compromised immune system is a major underlying factor in the development of FURD in older felines, all infected cats should also be tested for FeLV and FIV.

Depending on the severity of involvement, treatment of acute cases of feline upper respiratory disease may involve the administration of intravenous fluids to combat dehydration, broad-spectrum antibiotics for systemic use and for topical use on the eyes, and/or staunch nutritional support. This latter therapy is very important in cats suffering from this clinical syndrome because feline upper respiratory disease is often accompanied by a temporary loss of smell, an important appetite stimulant in cats. The loss in appetite that usually follows can quickly lead to malnourishment, dehydration, and fatty liver disease (see Feline Liver Disease, page 119). Nasal decongestants and room vaporizers can play an important role in helping to restore smell and stimulate appetite in these cats. Highly aromatic foods such as baby foods can be fed, or standard rations may be heated to help increase the food's aroma. If all efforts to stimulate appetite fail, hospitalization and force-feeding with a syringe and/or feeding tube may become necessary.

Prevention of upper respiratory disease is achieved using vaccinations administered either intranasally or by injection. Other methods of protecting cats against upper respiratory disease include limiting interaction with stray cats, maintaining a high plane of nutrition, and reducing stress within the environment. Because new cats, especially kittens, brought into a household pose the greatest threat to older cats, these new additions should be isolated for at least three weeks before allowing them to interact with the established house cat. In addition, good sanitation and hygiene on the part of an owner, especially following visits to other cat-owning households, is important to keep from inadvertently bringing a disease back home.

Feline Panleukopenia (Feline Distemper)

Panleukopenia is a highly contagious viral disease that causes severe gastrointestinal inflammation in affected cats. Caused by a parvovirus, the disease can prove to be quite deadly if supportive treatment is not instituted promptly. Although panleukopenia strikes primarily kittens and younger cats, older felines, especially those that are unvaccinated or experiencing some degree of immunosuppression, can contract the disease as well. Older cats are usually exposed when new kittens are introduced into a household.

Panleukopenia is transmitted via contact with infected body excretions, such as feces, urine, saliva, and vomitus. Upon entrance into the body through the mouth and nasal passages, the virus sets up housekeeping and replicates within the tonsils and other lymph tissue in these regions. The virus then enters the blood and spreads to other areas of the body.

Clinical signs associated with panleukopenia in cats include fever, depression, vomiting, diarrhea, and dehydration. Oftentimes, affected cats will have a hunched posture with their heads placed between their forepaws in an effort to relieve the abdominal pain. One of the primary effects of the parvovirus is profound suppression of white blood cell numbers within the body. As a result, secondary bacterial infections are always a threat, and can be a significant source of toxin production within the body.

Diagnosis of feline panleukopenia is based upon vaccination history, clinical signs, and physical exam findings. In addition, during the acute stages of the disease, laboratory analysis will reveal a marked decrease in white blood cell numbers within the blood, helping to solidify a diagnosis. Cats suffering from panleukopenia are treated with intravenous fluids, antivomiting medications, and antibiotics to prevent secondary infections. Treatment must be continued for five to seven days, allowing time for the white cell count to normalize and the immune system to neutralize the infection.

As with any viral disease, prevention is the best cure. Protection against panleukopenia is provided through routine vaccinations, as well as quarantining any new cat brought into the household for at least three weeks.

Feline Infectious Peritonitis (FIP)

Feline infectious peritonitis (FIP) is a uniformly fatal disease that can strike cats of any age, including the elderly. In fact, cats over the age of 12 years seem to be more prone to FIP than their middle-aged counterparts. Caused by a coronavirus, FIP is unique in that the damage that is caused to the cat's system is not actually caused by the virus itself, but by the immune system response

Many cats with FIP are also infected with the feline leukemia virus.

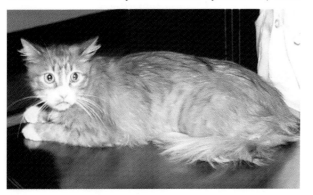

to the virus. In addition, to make matters worse, many cats infected with FIP also have a concurrent infection with the feline leukemia virus.

The FIP virus is transmitted from cat to cat via contact with infective body excretions or respiratory droplets. Because the virus is relatively unstable in the environment, close contact is usually required for transmission to occur. Once the virus gains entrance into the body, it infects white blood cells in the lymphatic tissue located in the nasal passages and oral cavity. Within a week after exposure, these infected cells enter into circulation and infect the liver, spleen, and other lymph nodes. The infection can also localize within the walls of the blood vessels, damaging the vessels and causing intense inflammation.

There are two types of clinical disease that the FIP virus causes in cats. The first type, called *effusive* or *wet* FIP, is characterized by effusions in one or all body cavities due to the intense blood vessel inflammation. With this type of FIP, abdominal enlargement is often seen, as well as breathing difficulties due to fluid accumulation within the chest and abdomen. The abdominal swelling is usually painless when palpated and as fluid buildup occurs in the chest cavity, the rib cage becomes noticeably incompressible. In addition, jaundice, anemia, eye disease, and gastrointestinal disturbances can be seen with this form of FIP.

The second type of FIP, called *noneffusive* or *dry* FIP, is the most severe form of the two. With dry FIP, small nodules and foci of inflammation are deposited among multiple organs within the body. Overt kidney failure, liver failure, blindness, and convulsions are all secondary conditions that can been caused by dry FIP. As the name implies, this type of FIP is accompanied by little to no fluid accumulation within the body cavities.

The FIP virus isn't the only coronavirus that can infect cats. The *feline enteric coronavirus* differs from the FIP virus in that, in most cases, it causes only mild disease with no apparent clinical signs. However, its significance arises when attempting to diagnose feline infectious peritonitis in cats. Because testing procedures available today cannot distinguish between FIP coronavirus and the feline enteric coronavirus, diagnosing FIP through laboratory blood analysis is less than reliable. As a result, veterinarians must rely on potential of exposure, physical exam and clinical findings, and analysis of any effusion that may be present.

Unfortunately there is no effective treatment for this devastating disease. Cats exhibiting clinical signs will usually succumb to the disease within eight to ten months after the appearance of symptoms. Both steroid therapy and chemotherapy have been used with mixed results in an attempt to modulate the immune system response in FIP-infected cats. Although such therapy is only palliative, it can help reduce the severity of clinical signs in affected felines.

Because there is no effective treatment, preventive measures against this disease are very important. Obviously, exposure to stray cats should be minimized. In addition, all cats should be vaccinated against the feline leukemia virus, because FIP is believed to be linked to the immunosuppression caused by this virus. In recent years, a vaccine has been developed and used in an effort to prevent the FIP virus from gaining entrance into the body. The efficacy of this vaccine, which is administered as nose drops, is still questionable. However, cat owners should follow the recommendations of their veterinarian regarding this vaccine based upon the relative frequency of this disease in their particular city or region.

Rabies

Rabies is a uniformly fatal disease caused by a virus that attacks the nervous system of its host. Cats, including older ones, are important carriers of domestic rabies; in fact, in recent years, the number of cases of rabies diagnosed in cats has exceeded the number of cases identified in dogs. The most common sources of infection in cats are bite wounds inflicted by wildlife such as rabid bats, skunks, and raccoons. Other routes of potential infection, though extremely rare, can be through the inhalation of concentrated, infective droplets or particles, or through the oral consumption of contaminated tissues or saliva. Following exposure, the disease may take up to 12 months to manifest itself outwardly with clinical signs.

Symptoms of rabies in cats can be quite varied, and may include behavioral changes, increased aggressiveness, excessive salivation, loss of appetite, restlessness, disorientation, pica (the desire to consume rocks and dirt), a drooping lower jaw, and/or generalized paralysis. Owing to the serious nature of the disease and the threat to humans, rabies should be suspected anytime a cat experiences sudden behavioral changes or neurological deficits. Conclusive diagnosis of this disease can only be achieved through a laboratory analysis of brain tissue from deceased or euthanized animals.

Because there is no effective treatment for this disease once it has established itself within the nervous tissue, prevention of rabies with vaccination is of the utmost importance. Another measure that can help prevent rabies is to limit exposure to stray or wild animals by keeping all felines confined indoors during the nighttime hours (see Vaccinations against Infectious Diseases, page 20).

If an unvaccinated cat is bitten by a known rabid animal, euthanasia is recommended to reduce the chances of human exposure at a later date. Vaccinated cats that are exposed to rabies should be given a booster rabies immunization and quarantined in an approved facility for not less than 90 days to observe for the development of the disease.

Any unvaccinated cat that bites a human must be humanely destroyed immediately and its brain must be tested for rabies. If a previously vaccinated cat bites a human, a ten-day quarantine in an approved facility is required to comply with most state laws (be sure to check with your veterinarian for regulations governing your state). During this time, if the cat exhibits any signs of illness, it should be humanely destroyed and its brain tissue should be tested for rabies.

Bacterial and Deep Fungal Infections

The bodies of older cats can become infected with pathogenic bacterial organisms secondary to invasive trauma, bite wounds from other cats, stress, viral infections, periodontal disease, allergies, parasites, drug therapy, and dietary indiscretions. As a result, whenever a bacterial infection is diagnosed, a thorough search as to its underlying cause, if not obvious, must be made as well. Bacterial infections involving the skin and tissues beneath the skin caused by wounds inflicted during cat fights are the prevalent types seen in felines. (For more information on bacterial infections and abscesses, see Abscesses and Bacterial Skin Infections, page 128).

Clinical signs usually associated with bacterial infections include depression, fever, loss of appetite, painful masses beneath the skin, swelling and inflammation at the affected site, and purulent (pus-containing) discharges. Blood work will usually reveal an elevated white blood cell count in these cats, although if the infection has been long-standing, the white cell count may actually be depressed. Chronic, recurring bacterial infections could have FeLV as an underlying cause; hence, FeLV testing should be performed on these individuals as well.

Specific antibiotics are chosen to treat bacterial infections based upon location, extensiveness, and the type of bacteria involved. Ideally, a bacterial culture and sensitivity test should be performed to identify the causative organism.

Older cats can also become infected with fungal organisms that invade deep within the tissues and cause intense pathological changes. These fungi usually gain entrance into the cat's body through the inhalation of fungal spores or by the introduction of the organism into the body through a wound. These deep fungal infections in cats include histoplasmosis, blastomycosis, coccidioidomycosis, and cryptococcosis.

The fungus associated with *histoplasmosis* is found in soil cont- aminated with the droppings of birds and bats. Gaining entrance into the body via inhalation of spores, histoplasmosis causes lesions in the lungs and airways, causing coughing and respiratory difficulties. From the lungs, the disease can spread to the intestines, leading to chronic diarrhea. Bone, eye, and skin lesions can also result from histoplasmosis.

Blastomycosis can also cause respiratory disease in cats, although it is rare. Infection can occur as a result of spore inhalation or wound contamination with infected soil. Other organ systems, including the lymph nodes, skin, bone, eyes, and the nervous system can become involved as well. Blindness, lameness, and seizures may result from such invasion.

Coccidioidomycosis is a soil-borne fungus more commonly seen in the dry, desert regions of the country. Infection usually occurs secondary to inhalation of spores from the soil. As a result, respiratory disease is the main manifestation of coccidioidomycosis in cats. Once in the body, the organism can spread to the bones and joints, spleen, liver, kidneys, heart, eyes, brain, spinal cord, and skin, generating related clinical signs.

Cryptococcosis is caused by a yeast organism that commonly affects the nasal passages of cats. The resultant rhinitis and sinus inflammation that occurs from such infection leads to sneezing, nasal discharges, nasal deformities, and

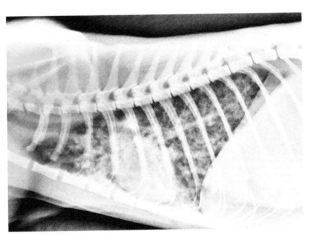

Deep fungal infection of the lungs as demonstrated on radiographs.

pose include amphotericin B, ketoconazole, and 5-flucytosine. These agents may be used alone or in combination with each other. If feasible, localized regions of infections should be surgically excised to speed a cure. When treated early in its development, a deep fungal infection can usually be managed and cured. However, if the infection has already spread throughout the body the prognosis is poor for recovery.

obstructive masses within the nasal passages. Cryptococcosis can also infect the lungs, nervous system, eyes, liver, spleen, heart, muscles, kidneys, lymph nodes, and skin of affected felines. Blindness, seizures, lameness, and draining skin lesions are just a few of the accompanying signs that can be exhibited.

Deep fungal infections are diagnosed based upon clinical signs, physical exam findings, laboratory blood tests for fungal antibodies, radiographs of the affected regions, and examination of cytology and biopsy samples obtained from the discharges or masses (granulomas) associated with the infection. Fungal cultures can also be performed on discharges and fluids obtained from lesions, yet these may take weeks to months to yield results.

Deep infections caused by fungal organisms require aggressive therapy, often lasting up to six months in duration. Antifungal medications commonly employed for this pur-

Internal Parasitism

Internal parasites can rob an older cat of much needed nutrition and weaken an immune system already compromised by age, predisposing the cat to other diseases and conditions. In addition, these parasites can cause vomiting, diarrhea, and dehydration due to gastroenteritis, and, in some instances, affect other organ systems within the body. Fortunately, diagnosis of an internal parasitism in cats is usually easy to achieve and, once identified, antiparasitic medications specific for the parasites involved can be administered to rid the body of an infestation. In older cats, internal parasites that may be encountered include roundworms, hookworms, tapeworms, protozoal parasites, *Giardia*, lungworms, and heartworms.

Roundworms
Roundworms, or ascarids, are thick-bodied, cream-colored worms

that inhabit the small intestines of affected cats. Existing within the lumen of the intestine and absorbing nutrients through its body wall, an adult roundworm sometimes grows up to 7 inches (17.8 cm) in length! If present in small numbers, they rarely cause anything more than mild intestinal upset; however, if enough worms are present, bowel obstruction, with its associated consequences, could occur. Immature roundworms can also cause damage to internal organs, because they may migrate to the lungs, liver, and other body organs, causing inflammation along the way.

Each adult female worm will shed thousands of eggs per day into the environment via the feces. Once consumed by a cat, larvae hatch from these eggs, and may begin a migration through the bowel wall and into the liver and lungs. Once they reach the lungs, the maturing larvae are coughed up and swallowed again by the cat, allowing maturation to be completed within the small intestines. Unique signs associated with a roundworm infestation can include a distended abdomen, vomitus filled with worms, coughing, and even neurologic signs if migration was extensive.

Hookworms

Hookworms are much smaller than roundworms, yet they can cause severe enteritis in affected felines. Instead of residing within the lumen of the intestine, these worms actually attach themselves to the intestinal lining using sharp mouthparts and suck blood and nutrients from this lining. A large worm burden within the intestines could lead to severe inflammation and irritation, not to mention significant blood loss.

As with roundworm eggs, hookworm eggs are passed out into the environment via feces. However, once outside, larvae hatch from these eggs and search out a feline host. They may be accidentally ingested by a cat, or they may bore through exposed skin in order to gain entrance into the body. If the latter happens, an intense itching and reaction at the site of penetration can occur. Once inside the body, the larvae migrate to the small intestines, where they reach maturity.

Unique symptoms associated with hookworm infestations include tarry or bloody stools, and weakness with pale mucous membranes caused by anemia. In addition, footpads and other regions of the skin that were penetrated by hookworm larvae can appear reddened, bleeding, and infected.

Tapeworms

Tapeworms are flat, segmented worms that can reside within the small intestines of cats. It is undoubtedly the most common intestinal parasite that will be seen in older cats. The most prevalent species of tapeworm in cats, *Dipylidium caninum*, uses the flea as an intermediate host. Tapeworm egg baskets that are shed in the feces of infected cats are consumed by flea larvae, inside of which they hatch into immature tapeworms and begin development. If and when a mature flea infested with a tapeworm is accidentally ingested by a cat during chewing or self-grooming activities, the tapeworm is released into the small intestine of the cat, where it attaches to the intestinal lining and completes its maturation.

Dipylidium infestations are usually easily diagnosed by the presence of white to tan tapeworm segments in the feces and on the hair coat just beneath the tail. As a rule, infestations with this particular species of tapeworms rarely cause significant health problems. Affected cats may have dull hair coats and experience mild weight loss, but diarrhea is rarely a factor with *Dipylidium* in the older cat. Treatment for these worms involves flea control and the use of antiparasitic drugs designed specifically for tapeworms.

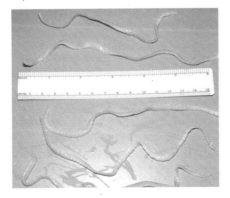

Tapeworms.

Elderly pets can harbor other tapeworms as well. These are usually contracted when the cat consumes raw meat or is exposed to wild animals. Unfortunately, these tapeworms are not quite as innocuous as the flea tapeworm, and can cause noticeable weight loss and enteritis in affected cats. In addition, many of these tapeworms can also pose a significant health threat to humans. As a result, if such a tapeworm infestation is diagnosed upon microscopic examination of the feces, prompt treatment should follow.

Coccidia

Another type of parasite that can cause disease in older cats is coccidia. Coccidia belong to a special group of microscopic parasites called *protozoans*. Transmitted from cat to cat by fecal-oral contamination, these parasites inhabit the small intestines and can cause diarrhea and dehydration.

Toxoplasmosis, a potentially serious disease in cats that can be transmitted to people, is caused by the protozoan *Toxoplasma gondii*. Under normal circumstances, most cats are spared from the clinical effects of an infection by this disease entity. However, stress placed on the immune system by certain viral infections, neoplasia, or chronic illness can pave the way for the appearance of a full-blown clinical infection. In fact, over 75 percent of cats showing outward clinical signs of toxoplasmosis are concurrently infected with FeLV. Symptoms and syndromes associated with toxoplasmosis can include pneumonia, gastroenteritis, fever, eye disorders, muscle pain and weakness, and inflammation of the brain and spinal cord. If the latter structures are affected, cats may exhibit profound neurologic deficits, including blindness, increased aggressiveness, weakness, and/or seizures.

Giardiasis

Giardiasis is a disease that may strike older cats and cause persistent diarrhea. It is caused by the intestinal parasite *Giardia lamblia*, a protozoal parasite like the coccidia. These organisms are transmitted through special cysts that are shed in the feces of infected cats. Once ingested by another cat via contaminated feces or drinking water, these cysts develop into mature organisms within the small intestine and can cause enteritis. Oftentimes, the diarrhea caused by *Giardia* is intermittent in nature. However, it does usually exhibit a characteristic yellow, foamy appearance when it occurs.

Lungworms

As the name implies, lungworms reside within the respiratory tract of affected felines. Fortunately, these parasites in themselves rarely cause severe clinical signs when they infest older cats. When they do occur, those commonly seen include weight loss, chronic coughing, and breathing difficulties.

Lungworms have an interesting life cycle, utilizing a number of intermediate hosts to finally get to their primary feline host. Adult worms lay eggs within the lung tissue, and the resultant larvae begin to migrate toward the trachea. They are coughed up and then swallowed, only to be passed out in the stool. The snail or slug serves as one of the intermediate hosts for this parasite. If the larvae are eaten by a snail or slug, they will migrate through the organism's tissues, maturing in development along the way. When a small rodent eats the snail or slug, the larvae are released and migrate through the rodent's tissues, eventually creating cysts within these tissues. A cat becomes infected when it consumes the infected rodent. Following ingestion, the larvae are released from the cysts in the cat's gut and migrate through the body tissues until finally reaching the lungs, where the cycle begins all over again.

Heartworms

Although heartworm disease is traditionally associated with dogs, its incidence in cats seems to be slowly on the rise. Caused by the same mosquito-borne organism that infects canines, *Dirofilaria immitis*, heartworm disease usually manifests itself as a much milder disease in cats. Because the cat is not the primary host of this parasitism, most cats harboring adult heartworms have fewer than ten adult worms residing in their heart, and show no clinical signs of infestation. However, in select cases, damage to the heart and other organs can lead to breathing difficulties, coughing, vomiting, and/or blindness. Older cats with preexisting heart disease are especially prone to developing clinical signs associated with a heartworm infestation.

Cats allowed to roam freely outdoors are at greatest risk of contracting this disease due to their increased exposure to mosquitoes. Testing procedures used to diagnose heartworms in dogs can be used for cats as well, yet because the worm burden in cats tends to be very minimal, infestations can be difficult to pick up in routine testing. As a result, many veterinarians rely upon clinical signs seen and radiographs for a diagnosis in these instances. If diagnosed, treatment for feline heartworm disease consists of hospitalization and administration of special medications designed to kill the adult worms.

Because the incidence of this disease is currently low, veterinarians are not yet recommending preventive medication be given to cats to prevent heartworms. However, the use of such medication could be warranted in the future if this parasite continues to adapt to this new host.

Diagnosis and Treatment of Internal Parasitism

Diagnosis of all of the parasites mentioned above (except heartworms) can be achieved through the microscopic examination of a representative stool sample. As a rule, the fresher the stool sample is when examined, the better the chances are for accurate results. In the case of tapeworms and protozoans, multiple samples may need to be tested in order to completely rule out an infestation. Diagnosis of heartworm infestations is assisted through the use of blood tests and radiographs.

Numerous effective medications exist for the treatment of the various internal parasites of cats. It is important to note that different medications and treatment regimens are required for each parasite mentioned. As a result, attempting to treat suspected parasitism without first having veterinary identification of the exact organism involved is futile and can be dangerous to the health of not only the cat, but the owner as well. In addition, these treatments should be performed only by a licensed veterinarian to ensure complete elimination of the infestation.

Prevention is the preferred method of "treatment" for any internal parasitism. Strict sanitation measures can help protect both the cat and owner from exposure to potential parasites. Disposal of fecal material within one day after its deposition will keep potentially infective eggs from contaminating the cat's environment. In addition, prompt treatment of any confirmed parasitism will also prevent this environmental contamination from becoming excessive. Complete flea control and prohibiting access to raw meat or wildlife will help keep tapeworm infestations to a minimum. Preventing feline interaction with wild rodents will help curb the spread of lungworms. Finally, supervision of a cat's outdoor activity will reduce the chances of incidental exposure to infective eggs or larvae.

The Cardiovascular and Hemolymphatic Systems

The function of the cardiovascular system is to transport oxygen and nutrients to, and carbon dioxide and waste material from, tissues and organs throughout the body. At the center of this system is the heart, a hollow organ with strong, muscular walls. The heart contains valves within its walls designed to keep blood flowing efficiently in one direction. From the heart, thick-walled, elastic arteries carry oxygen-poor blood to the lungs for replenishment, and the resulting oxygen-rich blood to the tissues of the body. Veins, which are thin-walled, carry the oxygen-rich blood that has circulated through the lungs back to the heart, and also carry blood from the body back to the heart after the exchange of oxygen, nutrients, and/or wastes has taken place at the tissue level.

The cells that make up the blood itself include *leukocytes* (white blood cells), a front line of defense against infections and foreign invaders; tiny cell fragments called *platelets*, which are required for proper blood clotting; and *erythrocytes* (red blood cells), which function to transport oxygen. Hemoglobin is the name of the molecule found within red blood cells that enables the cell to carry oxygen to the tissues. The noncellular portion of the blood contains water, nutrients, waste products, blood-clotting factors, and a wide variety of hormones, enzymes, plasma proteins, and electrolytes.

In addition to blood, lymph is a liquid material found within the body that contains immune cells (lymphocytes), proteins, and fat absorbed from the body tissues and from the intestinal tract. This substance is circulated throughout the body within special lymphatic vessels by rhythmical contractions associated with normal breathing and muscular activity. Eventually, after passing through many lymph nodes, which remove foreign substances and organisms from the fluid, the lymph is deposited into the bloodstream and reenters general circulation. In older cats, *edema*, or fluid retention within the tissues, can be caused by tumors or other disorders that block the normal flow of lymph through the lymphatic vessels.

Feline Cardiomyopathy and Heart Disease

Feline cardiomyopathy is a serious heart condition characterized by the replacement of healthy cardiac muscle with scar tissue and a resultant decrease in the efficiency and function of the heart. The exact reason this occurs is still generally unknown; however, genetics, certain nutritional deficiencies (taurine deficiency), and select medical conditions such as hyperthyroidism are thought to play major roles in the development of the disease. Cardiomyopathies tend to strike middle-aged to older cats and have a higher incidence in male cats than in females.

There are three types of cardiomyopathies that can afflict an older cat. The first type, *hypertrophic cardiomyopathy*, is typified by an abnormal thickening of the heart muscle walls, which prevents the heart chambers from properly filling with blood during normal circulation. This impaired filling, combined with the inefficient contraction of the thickened heart wall due to its size, fails to circulate adequate volumes of blood within the body, causing oxygen deprivation and damage to the organs and tissues. Interestingly, this type of cardiomyopathy seems more prevalent in Persian and Main coon breeds of cats.

The second type of cardiomyopathy is called *congestive* or *dilated cardiomyopathy*. In contrast to hypertrophic cardiomyopathy, dilated cardiomyopathy is characterized by a thinning of the heart wall and associated musculature. This thinning weakens the heart muscle to the point of interfering with proper contractions, leading to poor blood circulation. As a rule, the overall prognosis for a cat with this type of cardiomyopathy is poorer than those afflicted with the hypertrophic condition.

For years, the major cause of this type of cardiomyopathy was a deficiency in the amino acid taurine in the feline diet. However, because most feline rations sold today have adequate amounts of this amino acid either occurring naturally or as an added nutrient, taurine deficiency as a cause of cardiomyopathy has become much less common.

The third type of feline cardiomyopathy is actually a combination of both hypertrophic and dilated conditions. Such a combination severely weakens the heart and greatly interferes with its function, leading to dire consequences.

Not only can a cardiomyopathic condition lead to heart failure, it can also lead to the formation of blood clots within poorly circulated blood. In turn, these clots can cause a condition known as *arterial thromboembolism* in cats. Thromboemboli can occur anywhere in the body, and in cats, the sites most often affected are the hind legs. As blood flow is restricted to these limbs, pronounced weakness and pain results as muscle spasms occur due to lack of oxygen. The hind limbs of these cats feel cool to the touch, and a pulse in the legs is weak or absent. Diagnosis is based upon a history of existing cardiomyopathy and upon clinical signs exhibited. Prompt treatment of this condition with clot-dissolving drugs and/or surgery may yield improvement, yet the chance of recurrence remains great and the long-term prognosis is poor due to the secondary nature of this disease.

Clinical signs associated with feline cardiomyopathy will vary depending upon the severity of damage to the heart muscle. For instance, a mild case of cardiomyopathy involving minimal anatomical changes may only be reflected as a decreased appetite and a slight reduction in a cat's activity. On the contrary, extensive changes to the heart musculature can lead to the development of severe breathing difficulties as fluid accumulates within the lungs, abdominal enlargement as fluid is retained within the abdomen, extreme weakness due to oxygen deprivation, and, in advanced cases, shock. If thromboemboli are involved, mild to severe hind limb lameness or paralysis accompanied by severe pain may be noted as well.

Diagnosis of feline cardiomyopathy is based upon clinical signs, physical examination findings, and radiographs of the heart. Laboratory blood tests designed to detect insufficient levels of taurine within the body may be performed if such a deficiency is suspected. Further diagnostic procedures that are often performed to help determine the severity of the disease and prognosis include electrocardiogra-phy (ECG), ultrasonography, and angiocardiography. *Ultrasound* is an especially useful tool in distinguishing dilated cardiomyopathy from hypertrophic cardiomyopathy. *Angiocardiography* involves the injection of a special dye into the circulatory system, which then illuminates the heart and blood vessels allowing for easier visualization on radiographs. This procedure is used only in those patients who are stabilized and not showing signs of overt heart failure.

Treatment approaches are based upon the severity of the disease. Initial treatments administered to felines presented with acute clinical signs include drugs designed to dilate respiratory airways and increase oxygen flow to the lungs, diuretic drugs to mobilize excessive fluids out of the lungs and abdomen, and oxygen therapy. Specific cardiac drugs are usually prescribed as well, depending upon the type of cardiomyopathy involved. Their

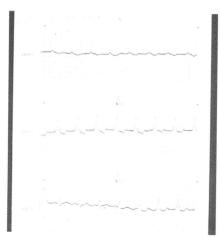

Electrocardiogram readings are needed to monitor older cats with cardiomyopathy.

purpose is to decrease the workload placed upon the diseased heart while at the same time increasing the efficiencies of the heart's contractions. In addition, aspirin therapy can reduce the chances of thromboemboli formation. It should be remembered, however, that aspirin is a very toxic drug to cats and should be used only in those doses and frequencies prescribed by a veterinarian. For those cases of dilated cardiomyopathy in which a taurine deficiency is suspected, supplements containing this amino acid are prescribed to counteract the deficiency.

Arrhythmias

An *arrhythmia* is a deviation from the normal rate and/or rhythm of contraction of the heart. When the heart muscle fails to contract in the proper sequence, or contracts too quickly or too slowly, poor blood circulation results. Arrhythmias in older cats can be caused by a number of underlying conditions. For example, weak, poorly timed contractions by the various chambers of the heart often accompany hypokalemia in cats. Also, *cardiac fibrillation*, an arrhythmia characterized by rapid, randomly timed, and incomplete contractions of the heart muscle, can occur secondary to hypertrophic cardiomyopathy. Urinary obstruction associated with feline urologic syndrome can lead to increases in serum potassium levels, and a corresponding slowing of the heart rate below the level needed for maintaining effective circulation. Hyperthyroidism, on the other hand, can speed the heart rate up so much that the heart chambers are unable to effectively fill with blood before the next contraction takes place, leading to circulation impairment and a worsening of the arrhythmia. Finally, poisonings, shock, and lung disease can all contribute to the creation of arrhythmias by causing electrolyte imbalances to occur within the body and/or by interfering with proper oxygen amounts from reaching the heart muscle.

Depending upon the type and degree of the malfunction, the effects of arrhythmias can be mild, causing few problems, or they can be life threatening. Regardless of the underlying cause, the symptoms associated with arrhythmias are similar to those seen with cardiomyopathies: coughing, weakness, breathing distress, weight loss, and exercise intolerance. Arrhythmias are diagnosed using a physical examination and an ECG reading. Treatment involves the use of antiarrhythmic drugs while the underlying disorder is being addressed. In severe cases in which an underlying disorder cannot be effectively dealt with, a pacemaker may be required for the long-term management of the arrhythmia.

Hypokalemia

Potassium is one of the most important electrolytes found within the body. Its primary functions involve the transmission of nerve impulses throughout the body and the contraction of muscle tissue, including that found within the heart. A deficiency in this important electrolyte within the body and bloodstream can have serious adverse health consequences. Unfortunately, the incidence of such a deficiency is quite high in older cats suffering from debilitating illnesses. *Hypokalemia*, or low potassium levels within the blood, is often seen secondary to kidney disease, liver disease, diabetes mellitus, feline urologic syndrome, and clinical signs such as anorexia, vomiting, and diarrhea. Hypokalemia can also occur secondary to certain drug therapies (urinary acidifiers, diuretics) and specially prescribed diets, such as those used to treat and prevent FUS.

Clinical signs associated with potassium depletion in older cats can include weight loss, weakness, lameness, muscle cramps, gait stiffness, mental depression, confusion, and breathing difficulties. An exaggerated flexion of the neck and head, caused by muscle weakness, may be seen in some advanced cases. In addition, weakness involving the smooth muscles of the intestines and bladder often lead to the retention of feces (constipation) and urine in affected felines. Low potassium levels disrupt normal electrical flow within the heart, leading to a slowed heart rate and abnormal heart muscle contrac-

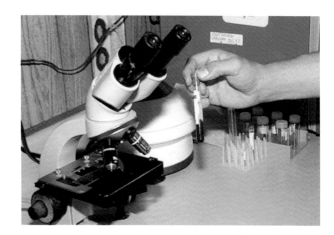

tions. This disruption in circulation can also adversely affect the kidney's ability to concentrate urine and rid the body of wastes, often exacerbating an already existing age-related compromise of kidney function.

Laboratory evaluation of blood serum potassium levels is used to detect hypokalemia.

Because hypokalemia usually occurs secondary to other disease conditions, clinical signs of potassium depletion can be masked behind symptoms associated with the primary illness, creating an extremely dangerous situation. If hypokalemic cats are not recognized and treated in a timely manner, death can result, usually from circulatory collapse or from paralysis of the muscles involved in respiration.

Diagnosis of potassium depletion in cats is made from evaluation of potassium levels in the blood serum. In normal cats, serum potassium levels should be around 4.0 mEq/L. Levels at 3.5 mEq/L or lower indicate a state of hypokalemia. However, such test results should always be compared with clinical

Table 15:
Causes of Potassium Depletion in Older Cats

- Anorexia
- Diets designed to acidify the urine
- Vomiting
- Diarrhea
- Kidney disease
- Feline urologic syndrome
- Diuretic therapy
- Insulin administration

signs seen, because normal blood potassium levels can occur in conjunction with potassium depletion elsewhere within the body. In these cases where clinical signs of potassium depletion exist in the presence of normal blood potassium levels, treatment should be instituted none-the-less.

Intravenous fluid therapy combined with carefully administered intravenous injections of potassium supplements are the primary modes of treatment in acute, life-threatening cases of hypokalemia. Close monitoring of blood potassium levels and ECG readings in these hospitalized cats is essential to ensure stabilization and to prevent serious health complications associated with an inadvertent overadministration of potassium supplements.

Long-term management in older cats prone to developing hypokalemia, such as those suffering from chronic kidney disease or recurring bouts of FUS, may include the administration of oral potassium supplements. Blood potassium levels should be checked every two to three weeks after initiating such oral therapy to assess dosage effectiveness. Following this initial phase, periodic blood tests every four to six months are recommended.

Anemia

Anemia refers to a total reduction in the number of red blood cells circulating within the bloodstream. Anemia can be further classified into either regenerative anemia or nonregenerative anemia, according to the body's ability to produce more red blood cells to replace those that are lost. Anemia in cats can result from one of three factors. The first of these is an actual loss of red blood cells from the bloodstream, which can be caused by internal or external hemorrhaging, parasites such as fleas, stomach ulcers, certain poisons, and internal organ trauma. Secondly, anemia can result from an abnormal increase in the destruction of red blood cells within the body and bloodstream. An example of this is the anemia seen with haemobartonellosis in cats. With this disease, the cat's own immune system filters infected red blood cells out of the blood and destroys them in an attempt to rid the body of the foreign invaders (see following). Thirdly, an overall decrease in the body's normal production of red blood cells can lead to or worsen an anemic state. Such a decrease can occur secondarily to nutritional deficiencies, kidney disease, liver disease, neoplasia, bone marrow disease, and viral diseases such as FeLV.

Anemia diminishes the amount of oxygen available for tissue and cell use; as a result, clinical signs of oxygen deprivation become most apparent. These include weakness, labored breathing, and an overall pale or white appearance to the gums and other mucous membranes of the body. In addition, in those instances where red blood cells are being destroyed by the body, the skin and mucous membranes may appear jaundiced as well.

Anemia can be diagnosed through the use of a laboratory blood analysis. Specific treatment depends upon proper identification and treatment of the inciting condition. General treatments for this potentially life-threatening condition include blood transfusions, oxygen therapy, antibiotics, B vitamins, and anabolic steroids. In cases of immune-mediated anemia, high dosages of corticosteroids will be needed to suppress the immune system and prevent further damage. High-quality, high-energy diets are usually prescribed to assist the cat's body in replenishing its supply of red blood cells.

Haemobartonellosis (Feline Infectious Anemia)

Haemobartonellosis is caused by a special type of bacterium that affects the blood of cats. In an active infection, *Haemobartonella* attaches to the surface of red blood cells within circulation. This, in turn, causes the body to react to remove the infected cells from circulation and effectively destroy them. This massive destruction performed by the immune system leads to severe anemia in affected cats.

Haemobartonellosis is seen primarily in male cats that are allowed to roam free outdoors. The disease is transmitted from cat to cat by blood-sucking insects, such as fleas and possibly mosquitoes. Clinical signs seen in infected felines include loss of appetite, weakness, fever, and pale mucous membranes. Cats suffering from especially severe immune system reactions may also exhibit vomiting, dehydration, and jaundice. Definitive diagnosis of haemobartonellosis is relatively simple, achievable through the microscopic identification of the organisms clinging to the surfaces of red cells within a blood sample. However, because of the clearing activity performed by the immune system against this organism, multiple blood samples may be need to be viewed before a positive diagnosis can be made. Cats diagnosed with haemobartonellosis should also undergo FeLV and FIV testing, because these agents are commonly associated with these infections.

Treatment of haemobartonella in cats involves the use of high doses of oxytetracycline antibiotics given over a three- to four-week period. In addition, corticosteroid medications can be used to prevent or reduce the destruction of red blood cells by the body's own immune system. Blood transfusions are indicated when life-threatening anemia exists. In especially tough cases that fail to respond to conventional therapy, thiacetarsemide sodium (the same drug used to treat heartworm disease in dogs) can be employed to help control this disease.

Unfortunately, felines infected with *Haemobartonella felis* can rarely be cured completely, even with intense treatment. Most treated cats become carriers of the disease and remain infected without exhibiting clinical signs. Relapses often occur when stress or disease debilitates the pet. As a result, prevention of this disease is of the utmost importance. Preventive measures against haemobartonellosis include stress control, vaccination against feline leukemia, discouragement of roaming activity and interaction with stray cats, and maintenance of a high plane of nutrition to keep the immune system working at optimum level. Control of biting insects using insect repellents and insecticides may also reduce the incidences of exposure to this organism.

Cytauxzoonosis

Like haemobartonellosis, cytauxzoonosis is a disease that can cause anemia in infected cats. Caused by a protozoal organism that is transmitted by ticks, cytauxzoonosis is endemic in the southeastern portion of the United States, especially in heavily wooded areas containing large populations of ticks. Clinical signs associated with this disease are related to the anemia it causes, and can include loss of appetite, weakness, breathing difficulties, and pale mucous membranes.

Diagnosis of cytauxzoonosis is achieved by microscopically examining specially stained blood smears. Unfortunately, there is no effective treatment for this disease, and it is almost always fatal. As a result, strict preventive measures, including tick control and limiting access to high-risk environmental areas, are a must in those regions of the country where cytauxzoonosis is known to occur.

The Respiratory System

The function of the respiratory system is to provide oxygen to and remove carbon dioxide from the circulatory system. Because oxygen is required for all metabolic reactions occurring within the body, unimpeded functioning of this system is vital to the continuance of life processes. In cats, the respiratory system also serves as the primary method of thermoregulation for the body, transferring heat with each exhaled breath. This system begins with the nose and mouth, and continues on with the trachea, a tubular structure composed of firm, cartilaginous support rings that help it maintain its cylindrical shape. After entering the chest cavity, the trachea splits into two bronchi, which branch even further into smaller units. The alveoli, which are formed by the lung tissue, are fed by these smaller units. It is here that the exchange of oxygen and carbon dioxide occurs between the lungs and the circulatory system.

Rhinitis

Rhinitis is an inflammatory condition involving the nose and nasal passages of affected cats. The symptoms usually seen with rhinitis include nasal discharges, sneezing, and gagging due to postnasal drip. Bacterial infections, fungal infections, nasal tumors, nasal foreign bodies, and trauma to the nasal passages are the most common causes of rhinitis in older cats. Oftentimes, infections associated with rhinitis appear secondary to disease-related immunodeficiencies or to immunosuppression caused by drug therapy (steroid therapy, chemotherapy). In long-standing cases of rhinitis, secondary fungal infections can arise. These infections are characterized by thick, mucoid discharges that may turn bloody if blood vessels within the nose become involved.

The underlying cause of rhinitis is diagnosed through the use of clinical signs, physical examination, radiographs, visual examination of the nasal passageways under sedation, and/or microscopic examination of the nasal discharge. Specific treatment will be determined by this underlying cause. In cases of infection, properly selected antimicrobial therapy will help bring the rhinitis under control. In addition, anti-inflammatory medications may be employed to help eliminate the clinical signs. All disease conditions that may be stressing and suppressing the immune system must be properly identified and addressed if the cure is to be long lasting. In select cases, surgery may be required to remove foreign bodies, such as grass awns or tumors that may be causing the inflammation.

Nasopharyngeal Polyps

Nasopharyngeal polyps are benign, pendulous masses that are associated with chronic ear infections in cats. These polyps normally arise within the throat region and extend into the back portion of the nasal cavity. They may grow to significant sizes and actually interfere with the normal flow of air into the trachea and respiratory airways, causing breathing difficulties.

Clinical signs associated with nasopharyngeal polyps in cats include noisy breathing sounds, sneezing, nasal discharge, and swallowing difficulties. If the polyps arising from the ear canal are large enough, vestibular signs including head tilting, head shaking, incoordination, and falling may also be associated with this condition.

Diagnosis of nasopharyngeal polyps can usually be definitively made upon visual examination of the oral cavity of cats suspected of having this disease. If diagnosed, surgical removal of the polyp is indicated; however, such a procedure is not without its potential complications. Because of the number of nerve fibers that course through the middle ear canal, surgical removal of polyps can lead to localized nerve damage, which can lead to side effects such as paralysis of the muscles of the face and excessive drooling.

Feline Asthma (Allergic Bronchitis)

Feline asthma, or *allergic bronchitis,* is a significant source of coughing and respiratory difficulties in older cats. The asthma attacks experienced by affected cats are similar to those seen in humans. The underlying source of the disorder is an allergy to some substance in the environment, such as cat litter, cigarette smoke, dust, disinfectants, and even something as innocuous as a feather pillow. Depending upon the inciting cause, feline asthma attacks may be seasonal in nature. They can also be brought about and worsened by stress. Allergic bronchitis is characterized by a constriction and narrowing of the respiratory airways, along with an excessive accumulation of mucus along the airway linings. Left unmanaged for an extended period of time, feline asthma can lead to permanent damage within the respiratory sys-

tem and lead to nagging respiratory problems as the cat gets older. Siamese cats appear to be especially prone to this disorder.

Clinical signs associated with feline asthma include a dry, hacking cough that may also be accompanied by wheezing and gagging. This cough may last several seconds to several minutes. Cats suffering from this affliction characteristically shrink to the ground and extend their head and neck in order to allow for easier passage of air into the lungs. Diagnosis of feline asthma is based upon these clinical signs, as well as ruling out other potential causes of coughing and gagging in older cats. These can include hairballs, heartworms, lungworms, pneumonia, and cardiomyopathy. Special laboratory blood work, combined with radiographs of the chest can help differentiate allergic bronchitis from these other disorders.

Feline asthma will usually respond quite well to treatment if properly diagnosed. Medications designed to dilate the airways to allow for easier passage of air, anti-inflammatory drugs to reduce the allergic response, and oxygen therapy if needed can all prove to be quite useful in the management of this condition. In recurring cases, long-term treatment with steroid anti-inflammatory medications can help reduce the severity of clinical signs as they reappear, and help prevent permanent scarring and damage within the respiratory airways.

Pneumothorax, Pulmonary Edema, and Pleural Effusions

Pneumothorax is a life-threatening condition caused by the influx of air into the chest cavity, either through a wound penetrating into the chest, or through tissue damage in the bronchi or lungs caused by trauma or by an invasive tumor. The resulting loss of the negative pressure that normally exists within the chest cavity can collapse the lungs and lead to profound respiratory distress. If this negative pressure is not restored in a timely fashion, either through the use of air drainage tubes and/or surgical repair of the hole or tear, death could rapidly result.

The accumulation of fluid or discharge, rather than air, within the chest cavity is referred to as a *pleural effusion*. Whereas allergic bronchitis may be one of the most frequent causes of coughing in cats, pleural effusions are by far the most common cause of respiratory distress and breathing difficulties in older cats. Effusions can consist of blood, pus, lymph, or a combination thereof, and can apply great pressure on the lungs, leading to the respiratory distress. *Hemothorax* refers to the accumulation of blood within the chest cavity. Trauma, blood-clotting disorders, and tears in the blood vessels supplying the lungs can all contribute to the formation of hemothorax in cats. *Pyothorax* denotes the accumulation of pus in this cavity. Bac-terial infection of the lungs or pleural space secondary to bite wounds from other cats is the most common cause of this type of pleural effusion. *Chylothorax* refers to the build up of lymph within the chest cavity. Chylothorax commonly occurs secondary to tumors and/or inflammation involving the lymphatic chain located within the chest cavity. Finally, pale to dark yellow-orange effusions of varying consistencies can occur in older cats secondary to diseases like FIP, cardiomyopathy, liver disease, and lymphosarcoma.

Whereas effusions refer to the accumulation of fluid within the chest cavity, *pulmonary edema* is the term given to the accumulation of fluid within the lung tissue itself. In this instance, respiratory distress is caused by lack of oxygen exchange instead of abnormal amounts of pressure placed on the lungs. The causes of pulmonary edema in older cats include cardiomyopathy, feline asthma, electric shock, neoplasia, pneumonia, trauma to the chest, and allergic reactions. Other less common causes of pulmonary edema in cats include aspiration of stomach contents into the lungs, and inhalation of toxic fumes.

Cats with pleural effusions or pulmonary edema exhibit breathing difficulties and show intense weakness, exercise intolerance, and peculiar stances or postures associated with respiratory distress. A conclusive diagnosis of edema or an effusion can be achieved through the use of a chest radiograph and through the use of a fine needle aspiration of the lungs and/or pleural space.

Pulmonary edema is treated by first addressing the underlying cause, and then, if needed, utilizing special drugs designed to mobilize the fluid out of the lungs. Cats experiencing breathing difficulties that are suspected of having pleural effusions should be treated promptly, sometimes even before diagnostics are performed. Treatment for pleural effusion involves minimizing stress and handling as much as possible, oxygen therapy, and removal of fluid from the chest cavity utilizing a needle and syringe, or placement of a chest tube. Once the cat's condition has been stabilized and the efficiency and ease of breathing has been improved, specific treatments for underlying causes can be performed. For instance, if a neoplasia is diagnosed, subsequent chemotherapy will often reduce the amount of effusion created by the tumor. Antibiotic therapy will prove useful in those cases where bacterial infections are promoting the effusion. Finally, in cases of chylothorax, surgically ligating the main lymphatic duct within the chest cavity will reverse this condition.

Pneumonia

Pneumonia occurs anytime inflammation or infection strikes the lungs. It is an especially serious condition in older cats that may already be suffering from oxygen deprivation due to cardiomyopathy or previous age-related degeneration of lung capacity. The potential causes of pneumonia in older cats can be numerous. Secondary bacterial pneumonias are not uncommon in cats that have immune systems that have been stressed by other illnesses, such as kidney failure or FeLV. Fungal diseases such as blastomycosis and histoplasmosis can stimulate granuloma formation within the lungs and create a severe pneumonia. *Aspiration pneumonia* is caused by accidental inhalation of food or liquid, and can appear in older cats with oral or esophageal diseases, or in those felines suffering from seizures or persistent vomiting. Lung inflammation can also result from inhalation of smoke and certain caustic chemicals. Finally, fluid buildup within the lungs caused by heart disease or neoplasia, and encroachment upon healthy lung tissue caused by tumor growth, can also result in a pneumonic state.

Clinical signs of pneumonia include persistent coughing, fever, weakness, and loss of appetite. A wide-based stance with the neck extended and open-mouth breathing may also be seen in these cats. Of course, the degree of breathing difficulty will be determined by the amount of lung tissue affected.

Definitive diagnosis of pneumonia and its underlying cause can be made through stethoscopic evaluation of the lungs at work, and through radiographs of the lung fields. In addition, blood profiles may be run to determine whether or not an infectious component is present. If a bacterial or fungal infection is suspected, a culture of respiratory fluid and discharge may be taken to identify the causative organism and to select an appropriate treatment.

Treatment of pneumonia will usually consist of antibiotic or antifungal therapy to treat any infection present or to prevent the appearance of a secondary infection, drug therapy designed to mobilize fluid out of the lungs and expand the airways to promote increased oxygen flow into the lungs, and, in select cases, medications aimed at reducing inflammation within the lungs. Intravenous fluids are also prescribed for those felines with advanced cases of pneumonia to help replace body fluids lost through increased respiratory secretions and to prevent existing secretions from becoming thickened as a result of dehydration. As a rule, medications designed to suppress coughing are not used in cases of pneumonia in cats, because this would only serve to slow the expulsion of mucus and other excess secretions from the lungs. Stress reduction and forced rest are a must if recovery is to be expected.

The Urinary System

The urinary system functions to remove metabolic waste material from the bloodstream and to regulate fluid balance within the body. It is comprised of two *kidneys*, which are responsible for filtering wastes out of the blood, and *ureters*, which transport urine from the kidneys to the *bladder*, where the urine is stored until voided from the body via the *urethra*. Another important function of the kidneys is to assist in the production of a special hormone called *erythropoietin*. This hormone stimulates the production of red blood cells within the body and indirectly regulates blood pressure. The anemia often associated with kidney failure in older cats can be linked to a disruption in the production of this hormone.

Kidney Disease and Kidney Failure

Kidney disease is one of the most common disorders associated with aging in cats. In fact, it occurs at three times greater frequency in cats over ten years of age than it does in their canine counterparts. Breeds especially prone to kidney disorders include Siamese, Abyssinians, Burmese, Main coons, and Russian blues.

Kidney disease can be manifested as either acute kidney failure or chronic kidney failure. *Acute kidney failure* is characterized by a sudden loss in function due to an insult from toxins (antifreeze), infectious diseases, trauma, urinary obstructions due to FUS, or other similar offenders or offenses (see Table 16). This loss in function is

Table 16:
Underlying Causes
of Acute Kidney Failure
in Older Cats

- Cardiomyopathy
- Shock
- Severe dehydration
- FUS urinary obstruction
- Trauma to the kidneys
- Ruptured bladder
- Toxins and poisons (ethylene glycol, certain rodenticides)
- Drugs (select antibiotics, chemotherapeutic agents)
- Ischemia (oxygen deprivation)

Elderly cat suffering from emaciation due to chronic kidney disease.

manifested clinically as lack of adequate urine production, intense dehydration, hypothermia, vomiting, shock, and unconsciousness. Fortunately, if treatment is instituted quickly and aggressively and the degree of insult is not too severe, in many cases acute kidney failure

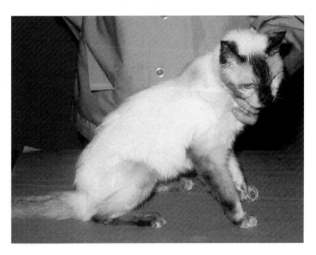

can be reversed with minimal residual complications. However, if treatment is delayed and/or normal kidney function cannot be restored in a timely manner, death can quickly ensue.

Chronic kidney failure is a nonreversible condition affecting the feline kidneys. It can appear as an aftermath to an acute crisis, as a result from wear and tear associated with aging, or secondary to a variety of clinical syndromes. One such syndrome that can affect older cats is called *glomerulonephritis*. This disease is characterized by inflammation and damage to specific kidney cells and tissue components caused by a unique immune system reaction to foreign invaders or other disease conditions within the body. In cats, FeLV, FIP, heartworms, pyometra, and systemic lupus erythematosus are just some of the diseases that can lead to the development of glomerulonephritis. Still another syndrome that can precipitate chronic kidney failure is *pyelonephritis*, a bacterial infection involving the kidneys. Oftentimes, these infections remain low-grade and deep-seated within the tissues, slowly damaging kidney cells and promoting scar tissue formation. Common sources of pyelonephritis include chronic, recurring bladder infections (which migrate up through the ureters to the kidneys), pyometras, and chronic periodontal disease.

As the kidney tissue deteriorates due to chronic insult, scar tissue begins to replace the once healthy kidney cells. As this deterioration progresses, the functional capability of the kidneys to rid the body of toxic wastes decreases, and they can actually physically shrink in size. Once 75 percent of both kidneys are negatively affected by this chronic deterioration, signs of kidney failure will begin to appear. Signs exhibited include depression, loss of appetite, increased thirst, and increased desire to urinate. Accumulation of waste products within the body can lead to ulcerations in the mouth, stomach, and elsewhere in the digestive tract, leading to vomiting and/or diarrhea. Oral ulcerations, combined with increased ammonia on the breath, cause a distinct halitosis in cats with chronic renal failure. Finally, anemia and its associated complications can also result from chronic kidney failure due to interference with erythropoietin production, and, hence, red blood cell production.

Definitive diagnosis of both acute and chronic kidney disease can be made through a series of laboratory tests performed on the blood and urine. By evaluating blood urea nitrogen (BUN) and creatinine levels within the blood and comparing them with the specific gravity of the urine, veterinarians are able to make a preliminary determination concerning kidney status. Under normal circumstances, the specific gravity of the urine, which measures how concentrated the urine is, should fluctuate depending upon the body's own needs for water.

Table 17: Underlying Causes of Chronic Kidney Failure in Older Cats
• Age-related wear and tear
• Toxins
• High blood pressure
• Glomerulonephritis
Idiopathic
FeLV
FIP
FIV
Lymphosarcoma
• Pyelonephritis
• Scarring from an acute kidney failure crisis

Diseased kidneys, however, are unable to conserve water for the body, hence, the specific gravity of the urine in a cat with advanced kidney disease will be low (dilute), even if the pet is clinically dehydrated and/or BUN and creatinine levels are high. If a problem is suspected, hospitalization for further testing may be required to determine the extent of the functional compromise. These tests may include radiographs, ultrasound, and biopsies. In addition, special testing to determine an underlying cause, such as FeLV, may be necessary as well.

Older cats experiencing acute kidney failure must be hospitalized and treated vigorously with intravenous fluids to correct water and electrolyte imbalances. In addition,

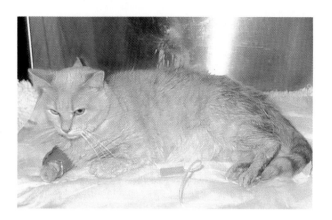

Older cat with kidney disease receiving intravenous fluids to correct dehydration.

medications designed to stimulate kidney function must be infused as quickly as possible. Urine production will be monitored closely, as will its specific gravity (indicating the kidneys' ability to concentrate the urine). If treatment is instituted soon enough, acute kidney failure can often be successfully reversed.

In the case of chronic kidney failure, the goal of therapy is not to reverse the condition, but to slow its progression. To begin, unlimited access to clean fresh water should be provided at all times to felines with kidney disease to satisfy increases in thirst and to effectively stimulate the kidneys to function. Withholding water from a cat with chronic renal failure for even a short period of time could be enough to induce an acute crisis. Secondly, special diets available from veterinarians should replace existing rations. These diets are specifically designed to reduce the amount of waste material produced during the digestive process, thereby helping to keep toxins at their lowest level

possible. Next, drugs to help regulate calcium and phosphorus levels within the body, anti-ulcer medications to help counteract the toxic effects on the lining of the stomach and intestines, and diuretic medications, such as furosemide, that work to stimulate the kidneys to increase urine output may all be prescribed to help alleviate clinical signs. In cases of long-standing kidney failure accompanied by prominent anemia, blood transfusions may be required to normalize red cell counts within the blood. Finally, an important key in the management of chronic kidney disease is to address any underlying sources that may be contributing to the problem. For instance, diseases such as periodontal disease must be addressed at the same time to prevent continued deterioration. Cat owners must also be cognizant of the fact that even mild episodes of vomiting and/or diarrhea can have profound effects on the water and pH balance within the body of older cats with kidney disease, leading to rapid dehydration and associated complications. As a result, prompt veterinary attention should be sought should these symptoms arise.

Feline Urologic Syndrome (FUS)

Feline urologic syndrome (FUS) is the most prevalent disorder affecting the urinary system of cats. Characterized by the formation of crystals and small uroliths (urinary stones) within the bladder that can nick and cut the linings of the bladder and urethra, FUS causes intense inflammation within the lower urinary tract, and can predispose the region to secondary bacterial infections. Both male and female cats can be affected; however, because the urethra of the male cat is much narrower than that of the female, the crystals and stones resulting from this disorder may coalesce and create an obstruction to urine flow in the male, creating a potentially life-threatening scenario.

The causes and predisposing factors of FUS are numerous. Stress, obesity, anatomical defects involving the bladder or urethra, and even certain feline viruses have all been implicated in the development of this disease. Bacterial infections are not considered an important cause of FUS in cats by themselves, yet when combined with other predisposing factors, such infections can certainly propagate and enhance an existing FUS condition. Also, nutrition plays a leading role in the creation (and prevention) of FUS. Research has demonstrated that diets high in magnesium and ash content can predispose a cat to urinary crystal formation. In addition, cats fed such a ration in dry form versus semi-moist or moist forms also have a higher incidence of this disease, simply because the minimal water content of dry food is less apt to encourage frequent urination.

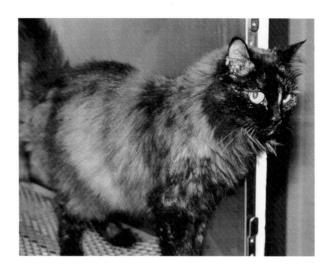

Clinical signs associated with an uncomplicated case of FUS include straining to urinate, bloody urine, frequent trips to the litter box, crying or vocalization during the urination process, continual licking or grooming on or around the urethral opening, and inappropriate urination in places other than the litter box. In complicated cases of FUS in which a urethral obstruction occurs, the clinical signs just mentioned are also accompanied by signs associated with urine retention. Despondency, vomiting, seizures, and shock can accompany those cases in which an obstruction to urine flow is present. These felines will have painful, distended abdomens, with grossly enlarged and firm bladders palpable in the lower portion of the abdomen. If the obstruction is not relieved in a timely fashion, irreversible damage to the kidneys can result.

Straining to urinate, and urinating outside of a litter box, are both signs of FUS.

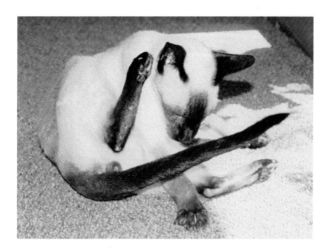

Cats with FUS may exhibit incessant perineal licking.

Diagnosis of feline urologic syndrome is accomplished using clinical signs, physical exam findings, and/or laboratory evaluation of the urine. Such urine will have a high (basic) pH reading, and usually contain blood cells and inflammatory debris, as well as numerous crystals. In addition, blood tests may reveal dehydration and elevated kidney enzymes in those cats suffering from obstructions. Radiographs may also be employed to rule out any anatomical defects that may be causing the condition. Finally, if bacterial infection is suspected, urine cultures are indicated to identify the organism involved and to select the appropriate antibiotic for treatment.

In complicated cases of FUS, prompt relief of the obstruction is vital to preserve the life of the cat. Plugged tom cats are started on intravenous fluids to counteract and prevent shock and to dilute any toxin buildup within the blood-stream caused by the urine retention. After fluid therapy is employed, a sedative is usually administered to calm the anxious cat and a urinary catheter is passed in order to dislodge and breakup the urethral plug. Once the obstruction has been relieved and the bladder emptied of its contents, it is then flushed thoroughly with a sterile saline solution to help remove any crystals remaining inside the emptied bladder. Because the chance of recurrence following this initial therapy is high, these cats are normally hospitalized and observed for three to five days, depending upon the severity of the case. The urinary catheter itself may be removed immediately following dislodgment of the plug or, depending upon the case, may be left in place for several days to ensure proper urine flow.

Uncomplicated cases of FUS and those complicated cases released from the hospital following relief from the acute obstruction are treated with drugs designed to relax the smooth muscle of the urethra and with anti-inflammatory medications to reduce the discomfort and severity of clinical signs. Antibiotics are often prescribed as well to prevent secondary infections. Also, medications designed to acidify the urine are used to help dissolve any existing crystals in the bladder and to discourage the formation of new ones. Special diets may be prescribed as well to help accomplish this latter goal.

For those cats predisposed to bouts with FUS, preventive husbandry measures should be taken by owners to reduce the rate of recurrence. The number one method of preventing FUS in cats involves dietary adjustment. Only those foods that are low in magnesium and ash should be fed to cats predisposed to this condition. As a rule, the magnesium content of a feline diet should not exceed 0.1 percent, with total ash content below 5 percent. In addition, the ration should also promote the formation of acidic urine, an environment unfavorable to the development of crystals. Fortunately, diets meeting all of these criteria are readily available from veterinarians and most pet supply houses.

Along with the type of diet fed, the frequency of feedings is also important in the prevention or encouragement of FUS. Following a meal, the pH of a cat's urine tends to experience a transient increase. As a result, those cats predisposed to FUS that are allowed to nibble on food throughout the day will have a higher average daily urinary pH than those fed fewer times during the day. Therefore, although feeding a healthy cat free-choice during the day is fine, those cats prone to FUS should be fed no more than twice daily, with any excess food being picked up after 30 minutes.

Providing a cat access to plenty of clean fresh water is another step in the prevention of FUS in felines. Encouraging water consumption by keeping the supply fresh will in turn lead to more frequent urination and have a flushing effect on the bladder. Most diets designed for the prevention of FUS contain increased sodium (salt) levels to stimulate thirst and do just this. In addition, feeding moist cat foods instead of dry varieties can provide additional water to the system and aid in thwarting the accumulation of crystals within the bladder.

In addition to changing the diet and encouraging water consumption, controlling and correcting obesity is a vital part of any FUS prevention program, because that condition is a major predisposing cause. Obese cats should be maintained on a reducing diet prior to being switched to a FUS therapeutic ration to help shed excessive poundage and increase the efficacy of the latter diet. At the same time, increasing the amount of exercise a cat receives will not only assist in weight loss and weight control, but will also have a tendency to increase water consumption and urination frequency.

Without proper management measures such as changing the diet, stimulating water consumption, shedding excessive poundage, and increasing exercise, the recurrence rate of FUS can be as high as 50 percent. However, it should be noted that FUS can also recur in a number of cats maintained on such a preventive program. In these instances, early treatment with anti-inflammatories, antibiotics, and, in some cases, smooth muscle relaxants can usually swiftly eliminate the clinical signs. For male cats that suffer repeated episodes of FUS-induced urinary blockage, a surgical procedure known as *perineal urethrostomy* may be performed either as an elective procedure or during an acute FUS crisis. This surgical technique involves the removal of the end of the penis and the subsequent widening of the opening of the urethra, allowing for easier passage of urine. Although this procedure won't prevent or cure FUS, it will help prevent life-threatening obstructions from occurring.

The Reproductive System

The reproductive system of the female cat consists of the ovaries (which produce eggs and reproductive hormones), the oviducts (where fertilization takes place), the uterus (the site of fetal development), the birth canal, and the mammary glands. This system can become a significant source of medical challenges in mature female cats that have not been previously neutered. Influenced over the years by repeated hormonal patterns, the reproductive tissues in these cats can experience abnormal anatomical growth or secretory activity. These changes, if significant enough, predispose the pet to several serious medical conditions. In older intact females, the uterus and the mammary glands are the sites of most troubles, if they are to arise (see Cancer in Older Cats, page 143).

The reproductive organs of the male cat include the testicles and associated structures, the penis, prostate gland, and two bulbourethral glands. Fortunately, intact male cats are rarely afflicted with reproductive disorders as they mature. However, they are not immune to neoplasia and other changes associated with aging that may involve one or more of these structures.

As a general rule, neutering at a young age or after reproductive efficiencies begin to decline should be performed to minimize these challenges. (For more information on this procedure, see Neutering Your Older Pet, page 35.)

Metritis and Cystic Endometrial Hyperplasia Complex (CEHC)

Female cats over the age of six that have not been spayed are susceptible to the development of metritis and cystic endometrial hyperplasia complex (CEHC). *Metritis* refers to inflammation involving the lining of the uterus, whereas *pyometra* refers to a condition in which the uterus becomes grossly distended with uterine secretions and inflammatory fluid.

The causes of metritis are numerous, and can include venereal transmitted disease organisms, endocrine disorders such as diabetes mellitus, abnormal pregnancies or births, and treatments with certain types of drugs. These drugs include hormones used to prevent or terminate unwanted pregnancies, and special hormones called *progestins*, used by some veterinarians to treat certain skin and behavioral disorders in cats. In addition, intact females become increasingly susceptible to CEHC with each successive heat cycle due to the hormone progesterone secreted as a natural part of this cycle. Over time, repeated exposure of the uterus to the effects of progesterone can cause the secretory glands within the inner walls of the uterus to undergo abnormal growth (hyperplasia) and secretory activity. This, combined with the progesterone's ability to decreases uterine muscle motility, can ultimately lead to fluid accumulation within the uterus. This fluid may escape out of the uterus in the form of a discharge. However, if for some reason it is not allowed to escape, a dangerous enlargement can result, with marked uterine enlargement, even to the point of rupture. Furthermore, the retained fluid can serve as an ideal medium for the growth of bacteria and other organisms, creating an infection (pyometra). In advanced cases, these bacteria and the toxins they produce can gain entrance into the bloodstream, causing blood poisoning. In addition, kidney failure can even occur secondary to pyometra due to the immune response mounted by the body in response to the infection.

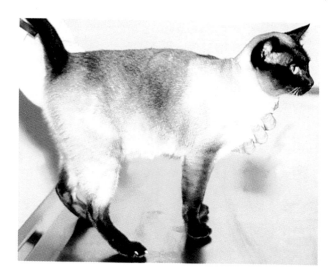

The most prevalent clinical sign associated with metritis is a thick yellow-green to hemorrhagic vaginal discharge. In addition, constant grooming around the vaginal opening occurs frequently with cats with metritis. In advance cases, loss of appetite, fever, and abdominal pain may arise as well. Finally, owing to the close proximity of the two organ systems in female cats, secondary bladder infections can arise resulting from metritis.

Cats with pyometra exhibit similar signs seen with metritis, yet a discharge may or may not be seen. Also, true pyometra classically causes a marked increase in thirst and abdominal enlargement in affected felines. If secondary kidney disease becomes a factor, dehydration, vomiting, or increased urination may be seen as well.

Diagnosis of metritis and pyometra in cats is made through the use of a history (intact versus neutered),

Older female cats that have not been spayed are at risk of developing cystic endometrial hyperplasia.

clinical signs seen, and laboratory workup, including blood tests, discharge cultures, and/or abdominal radiographs. In cases of pyometra, blood work often reveals a marked elevation of the white blood cell count and a mild anemic state. Abdominal radiographs reveal a grossly distended uterus that displaces other organs within the abdomen.

The treatment of choice for metritis and pyometra is neutering. Although select cases of metritis may be treated successively with antibiotic and fluid therapy, the chances of recurrence are so high that neutering should still be considered. On the contrary, pyometra in an older cat should be considered an emergency situation and surgical removal of the offending uterus should be performed as soon as possible.

The Musculoskeletal System

The *musculoskeletal system* of cats consists of bones, muscles, joints, and their associated structures. It functions to provide locomotory ability, as well as to protect and support vital internal organs. Accordingly, this system is designed to withstand enormous amounts of wear and tear that come with such important duties. Like other organ systems, however,

it is not immune to the effects of aging. These effects are reflected in a number of musculoskeletal disease conditions prevalent in the aging cat population.

Arthritis

Arthritis is technically defined as inflammation involving one or more joints of the body, with or without accompanying bony changes within the joints in question. Arthritis usually manifests itself as lameness and swollen, painful joints. In older cats, it is most often caused by abnormal stresses placed on a joint or anatomical anomalies caused by previous trauma to the joint. Arthritis can also be caused by infectious organisms invading a joint, or by an overactive immune system attacking joint tissue (immune-mediated arthritis). In each of these last two instances, fever, loss of appetite, and general malaise usually accompany the arthritic symptoms. Another arthritic syndrome seen in older cats is chronic progressive polyarthritis. This condition affects multiple joints in the lower portions of the limbs, causing pain and noticeable lameness in affected felines. The exact cause of chronic progressive polyarthritis has yet to be discerned, although certain viruses and even autoimmune reactions are thought to play a role in its development.

Diagnosis of arthritis is made through the use of a past history of trauma, clinical signs, physical exam findings, and radiographs of the suspected joints. If an infection is suspected, testing and evaluation of fluid obtained from an affected joint will be performed to identify the causative organism and to determine which medications will afford the quickest results. As far as immune-mediated arthritis is concerned, the most prevalent type seen in geriatric felines is systemic lupus erythematosus (SLE). Along with the arthritis it causes, SLE can affect other organ systems such as the skin, thereby assisting in a diagnosis. In addition, special blood tests and biopsy samples of tissue and fluid from affected joints can be used to obtain a conclusive diagnosis of this disorder.

Treatment of arthritis in cats that is noninfectious in nature employs the use of anti-inflammatory medications, including steroids, the strength of which is dependent upon the severity of the condition. If an immune-mediated arthritis is diagnosed, even higher dosages of steroid anti-inflammatories will be required for management. (Note: Remember that aspirin, acetaminophen, and other nonsteroidal anti-inflammatory drugs (NSAIDs) can be highly toxic to cats and should never be administered as a home remedy to suspected cases of arthritis unless specifically directed by a veterinarian.) Finally, treatment for infectious arthritis employs the use of appropriate antibiotics and antimicrobial medications, as well as surgical drainage and flushes of the affected joints in select instances.

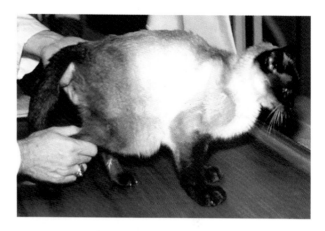

Testing joint mobility in an older cat suffering from arthritis.

Traumatic Injuries to the Bones and Joints

As muscle mass, ligament flexibility, and bone density are lost with advancing years or due to chronic disease, older cats become more susceptible to musculoskeletal injuries induced by trauma. Such injuries can include sprains and strains, ligament and tendon tears, joint dislocations, and fractures. Trauma associated with jumping activity, falling, and moving objects can usually be traced to injuries such as these.

Joint strains and sprains are caused by the abnormal stretching or pulling of the tendons and ligaments, respectively, of a joint. If these forces are great enough, an actual tear or rupture of these joint structures can occur. Obesity in older cats can also place a great strain on ligaments over time, predisposing them to injury. Severe strains and sprains, especially those that have progressed to a tear or rupture, usually result in a

Because of aging effects on the bones and joints, older cats are more prone to traumatic injuries caused by jumping from heights.

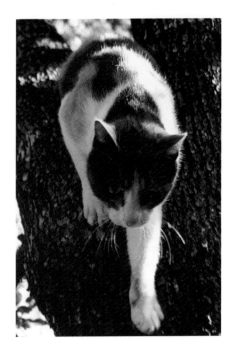

sudden non-weight-bearing lameness in affected cats. Within two to four days, function usually returns to the affected limb; however, a limp may remain. The joint instability that follows such injuries will eventually lead to arthritic changes within the joint and worsening lameness itself if the condition is not treated.

Diagnosis of a tendon or ligament injury is made upon physical examination and evaluation of joint stability upon manipulation. Radiographs may be helpful to determine the duration and the extent of the injury as well. Upon diagnosis, the treatment mode chosen will depend upon the severity of the injury and upon the weight and overall condition of the patient.

Initially, anti-inflammatory drugs can be used to counteract the joint pain and inflammation associated with the injury. Following preliminary treatment, surgical joint restoration is recommended in those cases of severe joint instability and loss of function. Many cats suffering these injuries may regain acceptable joint stability and function due to the body's normal repair mechanisms without any surgical intervention at all. However, the risk of arthritic changes in these joints occurring over time is still high if surgery is not performed.

Joint dislocations in older cats usually affect the hip joint, and usually result from a sudden impact imparted directly to the joint. Cats so affected will exhibit a non-weight-bearing lameness and marked pain involving the affected region. Diagnosis is easily made upon physical palpation and radiographic analysis. Due to the high rate of recurrence once a dislocation has taken place, surgical repair of the dislocation is preferred over the manual manipulation of the bone of the hind leg back into the hip socket. The surgical procedure most commonly used in these cats, called *femoral head and neck excision*, will eliminate recurrences of the problem and restore painless function to the affected limb.

Bone fractures are usually accompanied by swelling, pain, crepitation, deformity, and loss of function. They can be caused by direct trauma to a bone, repeated stress placed on a bone, and disease-associated weakening of a bone. Fractures are classified as either *closed fractures*, in which no portion of bone is exposed through the skin, and *open fractures*, in which one or more of the fractured ends of bones are exposed through penetrations through the skin, creating a high risk of secondary infection. In addition, they can be further classified as to the extent of the damage (complete versus incomplete), direction and location of the fracture line (transverse, oblique), and their stability following treatment (stable versus unstable).

Fractures are diagnosed based upon clinical signs exhibited and by radiographic analysis of the region in question. Management of the fracture will depend upon the extent of the break, its stability, and its location. Incomplete fractures that do not affect the stability of the affected bone(s) can be treated with pain relievers and forced cage rest for four to six weeks. Complete fractures involving the entire circumference of the bone and those fractures accompanied by instability of the bone will usually require surgical intervention in order for proper healing to take place. Open fractures will require antibiotic therapy in addition to surgical reduction to prevent secondary complications associated with infection from arising.

Most fractures involving the bones of the limbs, including the *femur*, the uppermost long bone of the hind leg that is a prevalent site of fracture in cats, can be stabilized with orthopedic pins and bone plates placed in or on the bone. Lower jaw fractures, seen secondary to automobile trauma and falls from heights, can usually be stabilized utilizing pins placed through the bones of the jaw as well as wires placed strategically around the lower teeth. Pelvic fractures may require pinning or bone plating if the fracture results in pelvic instability and/or the anatomy of the pelvic region and the pelvic canal (through which the colon, urethra, and reproductive structures pass) is grossly altered. Finally, fractures involving the vertebrae of the tail that result in nerve damage and loss of function to this structure can be managed by amputating the tail at or close to the fracture site.

Metabolic Bone Disease

Older cats that consume diets consisting primarily of meat or those suffering from kidney disease are susceptible to a metabolic condition known as *secondary hyperparathyroidism*, which is characterized by a generalized degeneration and thinning of bone. Elevated levels of phosphorus in the bloodstream can result from the high phosphorus content of all-meat diets or by the failure of the kidneys to correctly regulate phosphorus levels within the blood. These abnormally high levels disturb the proper calcium/phosphorus ratio in the blood, and stimulate the body to draw calcium out of bony tissue in order to reestablish the desired ratio. Unfortunately, the effect of this calcium draw on bone integrity can be devastating. Cats afflicted with metabolic bone disease can experience lameness, weakness, joint deformities, and spontaneous fractures associated with weakened and brittle bones.

Diagnosis of secondary hyperparathyroidism is based upon a history of dietary imbalance or the diagnosis of kidney disease, combined with the detection of elevated calcium and phosphorus levels in the blood. In addition, radiographic findings can be used to detect the bony changes caused by this disorder. Treatment of secondary hyperparathyroidism includes correcting the dietary deficit, managing any underlying kidney disease, and, in both cases, the administration of calcium supplements.

Another type of metabolic bone disease that can affect older cats is called *hypervitaminosis A*. This condition is seen in those cats fed an exclusive diet of liver, which contain high levels of vitamin A. Musculoskeletal changes seen in cats experiencing chronic vitamin A toxicity include bony deformities, outgrowths, and fusion involving the vertebral column, especially in the region of the neck, and bony fusion of the joints of the limbs, resulting in pain and immobility.

A history of an all-liver diet, combined with clinical signs and radiographic analysis of the spine and limbs can reveal conclusive evidence of hypervitaminosis A. If detected early in its development, this condition can often be reversed by switching the cat to a balanced diet. However, in advanced cases, the bony changes that occur are usually permanent, and anti-inflammatory medications are usually required for the remaining life of the cat to help ease the pain associated with the disease.

Myositis

When inflammation strikes muscle tissue of older cats, the term *myositis* is used. Myositis results in weakness and atrophy in the muscle groups affected. Affected cats exhibit pain upon movement; hence, they are reluctant to do so. In addition, when touched, these pets may vocalize or may exhibit aggressive behavior.

The causes of myositis in older cats can include trauma, infection, potassium deficiencies, toxoplasmosis, autoimmune disease, and poor circulation secondary to cardiomyopathy and/or thromboembolism. Diagnosis of the underlying cause is based upon clinical signs and laboratory blood tests designed to detect elevations in muscle enzymes and white blood cells. In those cases in which myositis is suspected, yet the blood work remains inconclusive as to an exact cause, a biopsy of affected muscle tissue is indicated as well. A cure, of course, will depend upon identification and treatment of the underlying cause. Antibiotics are used if an infection is present, and, in most cases, anti-inflammatory drugs can help reduce the pain and discomfort originating from the muscles. Myositis induced by an overactive immune system is treated with high doses of glucocorticosteroids or similar medications designed to suppress the inflated immune response. Finally, if poor circulation is to blame, concurrent treatment with drugs designed to improve blood flow to the muscles is appropriate.

The Nervous System

The nervous system is comprised of specialized tissues and organs designed to originate and transmit electrochemical charges to and from every organ system in the body, helping to regulate and coordinate bodily functions required for life, and to provide an environmental awareness. The main anatomical components of this system include the brain, which serves as the main control center for the entire system; the spinal cord, which acts as an information highway for nerves coursing to and from the brain; and nerve fibers, which interact directly with the tissues and organs. Groups or bundles of these nerve fibers coursing together are referred to as *nerves*.

Nervous impulses are generated from sudden changes in electrolyte ratios of sodium and potassium along the membranes of neurons, the cells comprising the aforementioned structures. These impulses then course down the nerve fiber until they reach its end. When this happens, special chemicals are released at the nerve tip, which transmit the impulse to another adjoining pre-determined nerve fiber, thereby keeping the impulse alive. In this way, a single impulse may be transmitted uninterrupted until it reaches its final destination.

The changes and disorders seen affecting the nervous system of older cats reflect alterations in normal nervous anatomy, slowed or incoordinated impulse transmission due to age-related degeneration, and/or disruptions in electrolyte balance at the cell level, which can occur secondarily to kidney failure and a host of other disease conditions. Keeping in mind the role of the nervous system, even the most minor alteration or imbalance can have profound consequences with regard to bodily function. As a result, prompt response to the appearance of clinical signs relatable to nervous system disease, including seizures, behavioral changes, weakness or paralysis, incoordination, and reduced organ motility or contractility, is advisable.

Feline Ischemic Encephalopathy (FIE)

Feline ischemic encephalopathy (FIE) is a neurologic condition that has been known to strike older cats. FIE is caused by a sudden disruption of blood supply to the brain, similar to a stroke in humans. Although a definitive cause has yet to be determined, cardiomyopathy, neoplasia metastasis, and even feline heartworms are suspect. Affected cats exhibit marked depression, incoordination, circling behavior, and/or seizure activity. The pupils of the eyes may become dilated, and blindness may be apparent. Acute clinical signs usually resolve within seven to ten days; however, residual neurologic deficits of varying degrees often remain indefinitely.

Diagnosis of feline ischemic encephalopathy is based upon history and clinical signs seen, as well as ruling out other causes of similar symptoms, such as vestibular disease, feline leukemia, and poisonings. Treatment of this neurologic disorder involves the administration of high doses of anti-inflammatory medications. In addition, medications designed to dilate the brain's

Incoordination and neurologic disease caused by peripheral vestibular disease.

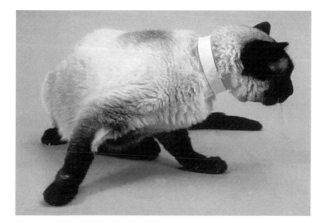

blood vessels and thin the blood may be employed in an effort to improve overall circulation to the affected regions of the brain.

The prognosis for survival in cats with FIE is guarded during the first 48 hours following onset of clinical signs. After 48 hours, the prognosis for survival is good, because FIE is a non-progressive disorder.

Peripheral Vestibular Dysfunction (PVD)

The vestibular system is a specialized portion of the nervous system found within the inner ear, brain, and spinal cord. Its duty is to maintain a state of equilibrium and balance. By communicating with the nerves supplying the eyes, limbs, and trunk, the body is able to coordinate the position and activity of these regions with movements of the head.

Peripheral vestibular dysfunction (PVD) is a disease that affects the nerves of the vestibular apparatus in the ears of cats. PVD is characterized by a sudden onset of incoordination and loss of balance, which is often accompanied by a head tilt, involuntary twitching of the eyeballs, and in many cases, vomiting. The causes of this disorder can include trauma to the ears, skull infections, and, especially in older cats, tumors involving the middle or inner ear. Diagnosis of PVD is achieved using clinical signs and various laboratory tests to rule out other potential causes of the symptoms. Radiographs of the skull may be helpful in the detection of any masses or infections that may be involving the inner portions of the ears. Treatment, of course, depends upon the underlying cause and usually includes high doses of corticosteroid medications designed to reduce inflammation involving the vestibular apparatus.

Feline Hyperesthesia Syndrome

Yet another neurologic condition often seen in felines is *feline hyperesthesia syndrome*. This disease has a pronounced effect on the overall behavior of affected cats. Siamese cats appear to be especially susceptible to this syndrome. Clinical signs seen with feline hyperesthesia syndrome include a marked adversity to touch along the skin of the back; in many instances, an actual rippling of the skin may be seen when touched. Excessive chewing and licking of the tail, hips, and flanks with subsequent hair loss in these regions is a hallmark of this disease as well. In addition to the dermatologic signs, hyperesthetic cats may suffer from hallucinations and exhibit strange behavior, often attacking inanimate objects and people for no apparent reason. In severe instances, these cats may suffer from actual seizures.

Diagnosis of feline hyperesthesia syndrome is based upon clinical signs and behavioral history. If diagnosed, treatment employs anticonvulsant medications and/or behavioral modification drugs,

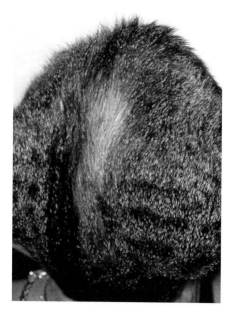

Neuordermatitis.

depending upon the severity of the disease.

Behavioral Changes and Senility

Apart from the obvious physiological changes associated with aging, behavioral changes may occur as well with advanced maturity. Changes in behavior most often noted by owners of older cats include decreased activity, reduced environmental awareness and alertness, decreased appetite, decreased social interaction, and alterations in elimination habits. Most of these behavioral alterations can be traced to diminished sensory function, decreased nervous system efficiencies, pain, and/or the effects of underlying disease (see Table 18). For instance, aggressive behavior in older cats suffering from arthritis, or

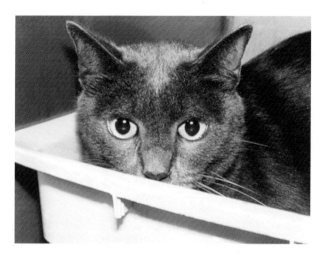

Behavioral changes in older cats can be caused by underlying diseases such as FUS.

even periodontal disease, can be sparked by even mild contact with the sensitive region. In addition, the appearance of a house-soiling problem in older cats may be due to senility, musculoskeletal weakness, endocrine disturbances, FUS, or dietary changes rather than actual willed behavior changes. As a result, a thorough diagnostic workup is warranted whenever a change in behavior occurs in order to detect or rule out any underlying medical conditions that may be causing the problem.

Diagnosis of a behavioral problem begins with thorough evaluations of its history, including time of onset, progression, and any distinct pattern of behavior that may have developed. Certainly a complete physical examination and laboratory workup is warranted as well to rule out any medical conditions that may be causing the abnormal behavior. Once such conditions have been ruled out, focus can then

be directed toward the management of the specific behavioral problem. Depending upon the diagnosis, such therapy may even employ one of several behavior-modifying drugs that have proven effective in cats (see Table 19).

Uncommonly, older cats can suffer from senile changes resulting

Table 19:
Select Drugs Used to Modify Undesirable
Behavior in Older Cats

Drug	Use
Phenobarbital	Tranquilization; excessive vocalization
Chlorazepate	Fear of loud noises
Diazepam and oxazepam	Appetite stimulants
Triazolam	Aggressive behavior
Chlordiazepoxide	Anxiety attacks; appetite stimulant
Alprazolam	Inappropriate eliminations
Acetylpromazine	Sedation, especially for traveling
Amitriptyline	Urine spraying; aggressive behavior
Chlorpheniramine	Self-trauma due to scratching and biting; sedation
Phenylpropanolamine	Urinary incontinence
Naltrexone	Self-trauma due to scratching and biting
Buspirone	Anxiety attacks; urine spraying

from degeneration of the central nervous system. Senility in cats is characterized by disorientation, confusion, and unfamiliarity with people and places with which they normally associate. Other signs of this condition include frequent pacing, repetitive grooming in a particular area of the body, increased vocalizations, alterations in sleep activity, and/or apathy toward life in general.

A number of conditions that may lead to the development of senility have been proposed. These include epilepsy, tumors, and other structural diseases of the brain that lead to a gradual degeneration of nervous tissue. Still another popular theory espouses that senility may have its origins in oxygen deprivation to the brain caused by heart and/or lung disease. Although all of these diseases and conditions may be suspect in the origination of this disorder, their involvement has yet to be conclusively proven.

Diagnosis of senility in older cats is achieved by ruling out all other potential causes of the abnormal behavior. Unfortunately, there are currently no approved drugs that are effective at counteracting the effects of senility. Certain management measures may be taken to comply with the decreased neurologic awareness. These can include altering the cat's environment in such a way as to allow for easier navigation, increasing the frequency of grooming sessions to make up for diminished self-grooming, and providing mental stimulation in the form of play and exercise on a daily basis.

Diseases of the Spinal Cord

The spinal cord serves as the source of communication between the brain and the rest of the body. As a result, diseases and disorders disrupting its normal function can have profound effects upon locomotory skills, sensory input, and internal organ function. The severity of clinical signs seen with spinal cord disease is dependent upon the extent and location of involvement. Early or minor involvement may simply lead to varying degrees of weakness and pain in affected cats involving one or more locations on the body. Cats with spinal cord disease may exhibit a reluctance to move not only due to these signs, but because of incoordination resulting from the spinal cord pressure and/or inflammation as well.

Hindlimb paralysis caused by spinal cord injury.

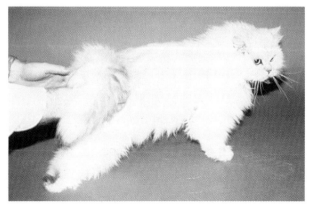

Extensive spinal cord involvements usually result in paralysis, loss of touch and pain perception, and/or internal organ malfunction or failure due to denervation. It should be noted that any spinal cord disease accompanied by any of the latter three of the signs mentioned above carries with it a poor to grave prognosis for recovery.

Trauma to the vertebral column and spinal cord is one of the most common sources of spinal cord damage seen in older cats. Fractured vertebrae resulting from encounters with moving automobiles, fractious dogs, or other sources can result in a partially or completely torn spinal cord in the region of the fracture(s). In cats, the lower back region is the area in which such fractures are most often seen.

Neoplasia and infectious/parasitic agents can cause inflammation and tissue damage in the spinal cord of older cats, leading to functional deficits. Lymphosarcoma is probably the most prevalent tumor seen affecting this structure, and classically causes hind-end paralysis. Feline infectious peritonitis is a viral disease that can settle into the spinal cord of cats and cause clinical signs of disease, as in rabies. In addition, the toxoplasmosis and cryptococcosis organisms can attack the spinal cord as well as the brain and eyes, creating a myriad of nervous symptoms.

Degenerative disk disease is one such disorder that can affect the spinal cord of cats. Separating the spinal vertebra of the back through which the spinal cord passes are special support structures called *intervertebral disks*, which serve as shock absorbers and points of flexibility along the spinal column. These disks are circular in nature and are composed of tough, fibrous tissue surrounding a gelatinous center. With age, a degeneration and subsequent hardening of this inner gelatinous mass may occur, reducing the disk's ability to absorb shock. As a result, affected disks become quite susceptible to compression damage caused by otherwise routine activities, such as running and jumping. Such damage can result in a rupture of the fibrous disk band and protrusion of the hardened center into the spinal cord space. Although in most cats such protrusions cause little harm, in some, enough pressure may be placed on the spinal cord to cause clinical disease.

Finally, *embolic myelopathy* is a spinal cord condition in older cats characterized by a disruption of normal blood circulation to the spinal cord. Cats suffering from cardiomyopathy and associated thromboemboli are believed to be the primary victims of this spinal cord disease. The paralysis associated with embolic myelopathy appear suddenly, and, depending upon the extent of the damage, may remain permanently in these cats.

Diagnosis of spinal cord diseases and disorders can be made based upon clinical signs, physical examination findings, blood profiles (if infectious disease is suspected), laboratory analysis of the spinal (CSF) fluid, and radiographs of the vertebral column. To pinpoint exact sites of spinal cord involvement, special radiographs called *myelograms*, which entail the injection of a special dye into the spinal canal, may be employed as well.

Treatment modalities chosen for spinal cord diseases are based upon the underlying cause and clinical signs exhibited by affected cats. Infectious or parasitic causes are treated with appropriate specific medications, if such medications exist. Spinal cord inflammation caused by trauma, disk protrusions, or emboli is usually treated with high doses of steroid anti-inflammatory drugs in an effort to minimize damage and speed recovery. In some instances, surgery may be required to repair a vertebral fracture, excise an offending tumor, or remove a diseased intervertebral disk.

The Endocrine System

The endocrine system consists of a vast network of glands and organs found throughout the body that produce and secrete substances called *hormones*. Hormones, in turn, regulate body functions and reactions vital for life, and coordinate otherwise complex interactions between the various body systems. Hormones are made of either protein, or of special fatty substances known as steroids. They are usually named according to their gland of origin (thyroid hormone), or by their action (antidiuretic hormone).

Both protein and steroid hormones are secreted directly from their parent gland into the bloodstream, where they circulate to the specific organ or tissue over which they exert their influence. The amount of hormone required for a desired effect is precise; excesses or deficiencies can lead to manifestations of endocrine disease. Such disruptions become more likely as a cat matures, simply because of normal age-related wear and tear on the endocrine glands, and because of the predisposition of older pets to neoplasia and immune-related disorders affecting these glands. In addition, because a single hormone may exert its effect on a number of different body systems and functions, any given endocrine disease can produce a wide variety of clinical signs.

Hyperthyroidism

A condition of hyperthyroidism in cats is caused by an increase in circulating levels of thyroid hormones, namely thyroxine (T3) and triiodothyronine (T4). When it occurs, hyperthyroidism is most commonly seen in cats greater than eight years of age, usually as a result of a tumor involving the thyroid gland(s). Because thyroid hormones help to regulate the body's metabolism, the clinical signs seen with hyperthyroidism can be directly related to the exaggerated increase in the cat's metabolic rate. These symptoms may be mild to severe depending on the amount of excess hormone being secreted. Signs typically include noticeable weight loss in the presence of a voracious appetite, nervousness and hyperactive behavior, and a rough, unkempt hair coat. Other less common signs seen include increased water consumption, regurgitation (due to rapid overeating), panting, and breathing difficulties, especially if the thyroid glands are grossly enlarged. In addition, over 35 percent of cats with elevated thyroid levels also suffer from inflammatory bowel disease (IBD). As a result, vomiting and/or diarrhea related to this may be seen in the hyperthyroid feline as well.

Diagnosis of hyperthyroidism is made through the evaluation of clinical signs, physical exam findings, and special laboratory tests. Upon physical examination, nodules can usually be palpated in the neck region due to the glandular enlargements. In addition, a rapid heart rate and pulse is often detected due to the thyroid hormone's affect upon the heart. This cardiac affect can be especially dangerous in older cats suffering from concurrent cardiomyopathy. Also, diagnosis of hyperthyroidism can be verified through the use of special tests designed to detect levels of thyroid hormone in the blood.

If this condition is definitively diagnosed, a number of treatment options exist. The type of treatment chosen will be dependent on the severity of the thyroid hormone elevation and on other underlying disease factors (such as the presence of a cardiomyopathic condition or kidney disease). Medical treatment for hyperthyroidism involves the administration of special drugs designed to inhibit production of thyroid hormone by the thyroid glands, thereby controlling clinical signs. Two of the most popular medications used for this purpose include methimazole and propylthiouracil. Side effects from giving these drugs can include anemia, immune cell suppression, decreased appetite, vomiting, weakness, and itching. Because most cats must stay on this medication for the remainder of their lives, close monitoring by and periodic communication with a veterinarian is essential.

Yet another form of medical therapy that yields very successful results in hyperthyroid felines is called *radioactive iodine therapy*. This type of therapy selectively destroys malfunctioning thyroid cells using radiation. Unfortunately, due to government regulations concerning radiation, this type of therapy is generally not readily available at most veterinary offices and hospitals. However, it is being employed at most veterinary schools and teaching hospitals across the country, and can be recommended on a referral basis.

Most cats suffering from hyperthyroidism will respond favorably to medical therapy. However if drug therapy fails to resolve the disorder and radioactive iodine therapy is unavailable, surgical removal of one or both thyroid glands (partial or complete thyroidectomy) must be performed. If extensive tumor involvement necessitates the removal of both glands, then daily thyroid hormone supplementation will be required for the remainder of the cat's life. Felines placed on such supplementation should have blood thyroid levels checked every six to eight months to ensure that adequate levels are being given.

An inherent risk associated with the surgical removal of both thyroid glands in cats is a complication known as *hypoparathyroidism*. This condition, characterized by low blood calcium levels, is caused by the inadvertent removal of the parathyroid glands (which are very small and tightly adhered to the thyroid glands) when the thyroid tissue is removed. Signs of low blood calcium, which normally arise within three days of parathyroid gland removal, include profound weakness, muscle tremors and spasms, and in some cases, seizures. Felines suffering from this postsurgical complication require prompt treatment with calcium supplements. These supplements, as well as vitamin D tablets, will be required for life to help maintain proper calcium levels within the body.

Hyperadrenocorticism (Cushing's Disease)

Hyperadrenocorticism is a relatively uncommon disease in cats characterized by an overproduction of glucocorticosteroid hormones by the adrenal glands. These hormones serve to regulate the utilization of carbohydrates, proteins, and fats within the body. In addition, they play an important role in maintaining water and electrolyte balance through their influence upon the kidneys. Finally, certain types of these hormones exhibit potent anti-inflammatory properties, a characteristic exploited by veterinarians for the treatment of feline allergies and inflammatory conditions.

In Cushing's disease, the overproduction of glucocorticosteroids usually occurs due to excessive stimulation of the adrenal glands by the pituitary gland. Tumors involving the adrenal glands can also lead to increased steroid hormone production. Clinical signs seen as a result include noticeable increases in food and water consumption, increased urination frequency, exercise intolerance, hair loss, dry seborrhea, skin pigmentation, and a diminished muscle mass and tone throughout the body. Ulcerations of the corneas of the eyes may appear as the disease progresses, and because high doses of certain types of corticosteroids can be immunosuppressive, secondary infections involving the skin and urinary bladder are not at all uncommon. If a tumor of the pituitary gland is the cause of the increased pituitary gland activity, seizures and other neurological signs may gradually appear as the tumor slowly increases in size.

Conclusive diagnosis of feline Cushing's disease can be made using blood tests specific for this disorder. In addition, radiographs may reveal adrenal gland lesions, helping to confirm a diagnosis. Treatment typically involves the use of chemotherapy to reduce the amount of steroids being produced by the adrenal glands. During the initial weeks of treatment, close monitoring for adverse reactions to the chemotherapeutic drugs is required. In conjunction with this treatment, antibiotic therapy may be prescribed to combat secondary bacterial infections. Lastly, surgical intervention may be attempted in those cases that fail to respond to medical management.

Hypoadrenocorticism (Addison's Disease)

Hypoadrenocorticism is in effect the opposite of Cushing's disease, with inadequate amounts of corticosteroids being produced by the body. Special types of corticosteroids, called *mineralocorticoids*, are vital to the maintenance of fluid and electrolyte balance within the body. Deficiencies in these hormones, as seen with Addison's disease, can create serious consequences.

Tumors, infections, autoimmune diseases, and toxins can all predispose to primary Addison's disease in older cats. However, most cases of Addison's' disease in felines occur secondary to the indiscriminate, long-term administration of glucocorticosteroids or other similar hormones to cats with skin or behavioral disorders. Such administration suppresses the adrenal glands' own ability to produce corticosteroids, including mineralocorticoids. As a result, when such therapy is abruptly halted, hypoadrenocorticism can occur.

Clinical signs in affected cats include loss of appetite, weight loss, vomiting, diarrhea, and dehydration. Profound weakness occurs as disruptions in sodium and potassium balance within the body lead to heart and muscle fatigue. In severe instances, the heart rate may slow to such an extent as circulatory collapse and shock could result.

Definitive diagnosis of Addison's disease is achieved by evaluating the ratio of sodium to potassium in the blood. Obvious increases in potassium levels with commitment decreases in sodium levels, in the presence of clinical signs and electrocardiogram analysis, is diagnostic for Addison's disease.

If history and clinical signs indicate Addison's disease, treatment should be started immediately, even before a final diagnosis has been achieved. Treatments with intravenous fluids and mineralocorticosteroids will be used to normalize fluid and electrolyte levels within the body. Once stabilized, periodic injections with mineralocorticoids will be required for life for those cats afflicted with primary Addison's disease. For those cats exhibiting Addisonian signs due to an abrupt cessation of corticosteroid therapy, reinstituting such therapy, and then gradually tapering the dosage given over three to four months to give the adrenal glands time to start producing their own hormone again should help prevent a recurrence of the crisis.

Diabetes Mellitus

Insulin is the hormone produced by the pancreas that is primarily responsible for regulating the utilization of glucose by the cells of the body. If production of this hormone is interfered with due to disease or injury involving the pancreas, diabetes mellitus occurs. Older, overweight cats seem to be at greater risk of developing this disease.

Clinical signs associated with diabetes mellitus result from the inability of the cells of the body to receive energy in the form of glucose. High levels of glucose in the bloodstream spill over into the urine, leading to increased urinations and thirst. Excess glucose in the blood can also infiltrate the lens of the eyes, leading to cataracts and blindness. Diabetes mellitus can reduce the body's resistance to infection, and affected cats often suffer from secondary bacterial infections of the skin and urinary tract. Damage to small blood vessels caused by the

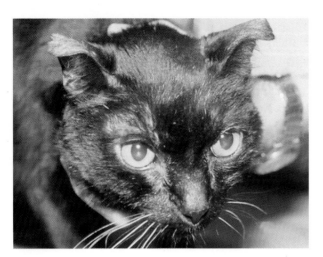

Cataracts and skin lesions associated with diabetes mellitus.

strating consistently elevated glucose levels in the blood and urine, and ruling out other causes of similar clinical signs, such as Cushing's disease and kidney disease. It should be noted, however, that not all cases of diabetes mellitus in cats are permanent. Many are transient in nature, lasting for several weeks or months before resolving on their own.

Treatment of diabetic cats suffering from severe clinical signs includes hospitalization with intravenous fluid therapy, blood pH modifiers, and insulin infusions. Close monitoring is required to ensure that blood glucose levels don't fall too low as a result of the insulin administration, leading to convulsions.

For those cats exhibiting uncomplicated signs of diabetes mellitus, insulin injections are indicated to help normalize glucose utilization within the body. Such treatment, which can be administered at home, must be performed in strict accordance with the treatment protocol formulated by the attending veterinarian. Depending upon the type of insulin prescribed, injections may be required once or twice daily. Accurate daily records reflecting morning urine glucose values as determined by special test strips, insulin amounts given, appetite characteristics, exercise activity, and any behavioral abnormalities must be kept. In addition, a strict feeding schedule should be followed utilizing special diets pre-

effects of the insulin deficiency can lead to kidney disease and gangrene of the skin and outermost extremities. Finally, in response to the lack of available glucose, protein and fat reserves are called upon by the cells of the body for conversion into energy. This often leads to profound weight loss and muscle atrophy. As fats are broken down for energy, substances called *ketones* are produced and accumulate within the body. If levels of ketones become too elevated, liver damage, pronounced nervous system depression, and pH imbalances can result. Cats with such severe, complicated cases of diabetes mellitus may exhibit vomiting, diarrhea, breathing difficulties, dehydration, and depression to the point of unconsciousness. Cases exhibiting such symptoms should be considered medical emergencies and treated accordingly.

Diagnosis of diabetes mellitus is based upon clinical signs, demon-

scribed for diabetic cats. Diabetic cats that are overweight will need to reduce as well in order to ensure maximum insulin effectiveness.

When administering insulin injections to a diabetic pet, begin by gently swirling the insulin vial to mix the contents. Do not shake the vial; to do so could damage the insulin molecules within the solution. Next, swab the injection top of the vial with a cotton ball and alcohol, and then using the insulin needle and syringe, withdraw the desired amount of insulin from the vial. Once the proper dosage has been prepared, lift or "tent" the skin over either shoulder or hip region. Firmly insert the needle into the skin and underlying tissue, using care not to penetrate the opposite side of the skin. Once the needle is inserted, withdraw slightly on the plunger. If no blood is noted, administer the injection and withdraw the needle. Dispose of the needle and syringe properly.

Be aware that injecting a deficient dose of insulin is better than administering too much. If too much insulin is indeed given, a condition known as insulin shock could result. Clinical signs seen with this condition are related to low blood sugar (hypoglycemia) and can include trembling, weakness, incoordination, and, in advanced cases, seizures. Chances are that if treatment instructions are closely adhered to, severe insulin should not be a problem. In some instances, low blood sugar can occur in cases of transient

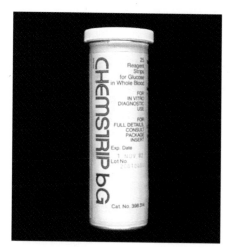

Blood glucose levels must be monitored closely in cats with diabetes mellitus.

diabetes mellitus that resolve, yet insulin injections are continued. To be safe, pancake syrup or honey should always be kept available for quick oral administration should signs of insulin shock begin to appear. Two tablespoons of either should be enough to replenish blood sugar levels and dissipate the signs of shock. No further insulin should be given following a hypoglycemic attack until veterinary consultation is received.

Hyperparathyroidism

The parathyroid glands, which are closely associated with the thyroid glands in cats, produce a hormone that is responsible for increasing calcium levels in the blood by drawing stores of this mineral from bone and other regions of the body. Hyperparathyroidism is a condition initiated by a deficiency of calcium within the bloodstream. This can result from feeding diets that are high in phosphorus (nutritional hyperparathyroidism), such as organ meat diets, or, more commonly in older cats, from increased phosphorus levels in the body caused by kidney disease. When such a calcium deficiency occurs, the parathyroid glands respond by secreting large amounts of hormone, which draws calcium out of bone in an attempt to normalize blood calcium levels. Over time, these bones become weakened and prone to stress injury.

Clinical signs of this metabolic disease in older cats include lameness, weakness, bone deformities, and spontaneous fractures. A conclusive diagnosis can be made by evaluating blood calcium levels and relating them to historical or other laboratory findings (history of poor diet, laboratory evidence of kidney disease). Treatment for nutritional hyperparathyroidism includes dietary modification and calcium supplementation. Unfortunately, there is no effective treatment for hyperparathyroidism caused by kidney disease except for treatment of the kidney disease itself.

The Digestive System

The digestive system functions to convert food into essential nutrients needed by the body for growth, maintenance, and repair. It also provides a means of eliminating waste material from the body. The organs of the digestive system begin with the teeth, tongue, and salivary glands. Chewed food is directed by the tongue to the esophagus, a long muscular tube that moves food down into the stomach through a series of muscular contractions. In the stomach, food is mixed with acids and enzymes to further continue the process of digestion. From the stomach, food enters into the small intestine, where special enzymes complete the digestion of foodstuffs into smaller nutrients that can be absorbed into the body. Undigested waste is then shunted into the large intestine, or colon, where water is either added to or reabsorbed from the waste material. Finally, it is expelled through the rectum and anus, thereby completing the digestive cycle.

In addition to the organs mentioned, accessory digestive organs that produce and/or store enzymes, acids, and hormones essential to the digestive process exist and include the pancreas, the liver, and the gall bladder.

Periodontal Disease

Periodontal disease is probably the most prevalent health disorder affecting older cats today. Characterized by tender, swollen gums, halitosis (bad breath), excessive salivation, and tooth loss, *periodontal disease*, if left untreated, can cause disease in other organs of the body, including the heart and kidneys.

Periodontal disease originates with the accumulation of food particles and bacteria on the tooth surfaces. This accumulation, commonly known as plaque, eventually mineralizes, forming a hard dental calculus on the surface of the tooth. Appearing as brown to yellow crusts, these calculi may extend up under the gum line, creating gum inflammation and pain. Left untreated, the inflammation and infection associated with periodontal disease will weaken tooth support structures and lead to tooth loss.

The type of diet fed to a cat can play an important role in development of plaque and subsequent periodontal disease. Older cats fed dry cat foods will be less susceptible to this disease than cats fed moist or semimoist rations, due to the increased sugar content of the latter types. Furthermore, diets containing excessive phosphorus, such as those consisting primarily of meat and meat by-products, have also been linked to this disorder. Endocrine diseases such as diabetes mellitus can lead to gingivitis and subsequent periodontal disease. Tumors involving the gum and/or base of the tooth or skull in the facial region can also play a role in the development of this disease. Infectious diseases such as FeLV and FIV can lead to chronic inflammation of the gums in afflicted cats and prepare the way for secondary bacterial infections. Finally, any disease that weakens the immune system and causes undo stress can predispose a cat to tooth and gum disease.

The effects of periodontal disease, in addition to those mentioned earlier, can progress to gagging or retching as inflammation peaks within the mouth. Gum recession, bleeding, and tooth loss arise as the disease reaches advanced stages. Infected teeth can form abscesses and can lead to secondary sinus infections, characterized by subsequent nasal discharges or draining tracks appearing on the sides of the face. To make matters worse, bacteria from infected teeth and gums can gain entrance into the bloodstream and seed the body with infectious organisms, affecting the heart, liver, kidneys, and other organs.

Treatment of periodontal disease is achieved through professional scaling and polishing the teeth while the cat is under anesthesia (see Dental Care, page 34). This procedure is essential to remove the calculus from under the gum line and to relieve any pockets of pus that may have formed near the base of the teeth. In addition, teeth that are excessively loose may form a nidus for infection, and are generally removed to allow for drainage and medication. Cats suffering from moderate to advanced cases of periodontal disease are also placed on antibiotics to combat bacteria that may have spread within the body as a result of the disease.

Plasma Cell Gingivitis

Plasma cell gingivitis is an uncommon disease affecting the

oral cavity of older cats. Character- ized by red, friable gums that often grow over and partially cover the teeth, this disorder leads to difficul- ties in chewing food, foul-smelling breath, and periodontal disease. Inflammation associated with the disease can also spread to the back of the throat, making swallow- ing difficult.

The cause of plasma cell gingivi- tis in cats is unknown; however, any insult causing chronic inflam- mation in the oral cavity could pre- dispose to this condition. Diagnosis is based upon biopsy findings of samples taken from affected tissue. Treatment involves surgical removal and/or cauterizing of the excessive gum proliferations. Steroid anti- inflammatory medications can be used as well to control associated swelling and inflammation. Unfortu- nately, recurrences of this disease are common, even after treatment.

Esophagitis

Inflammation involving the esophagus is termed *esophagitis*. Esophagitis is relatively rare in older cats, and when it occurs, is most often instigated by swallowed for- eign bodies that injure the organ's lining, by the accidental ingestion of caustic substances, or by reflux of stomach contents and acids up into the esophagus, such as that seen with chronic bouts of vomiting, associated kidney disease, and other conditions in older cats. The hallmark clinical sign associated with esophageal inflammation is the passive regurgitation of food and water. In *passive regurgitation*, digestive contents are expelled rather suddenly and uneventfully, differing from the abdominal heav- ing, gagging, and forceful expulsion seen with vomiting. If esophagitis is not addressed in a timely manner, damage to the lining of the esopha- gus can occur, causing strictures. This damage can also interfere with the esophagus's ability to contract properly, leading to a gross disten- sion of the organ with accumulated food and water (megaesophagus).

Diagnosis of esophagitis is made using clinical signs, physical exam findings, and radiographs of the esophagus using barium to high- light the organ's lining. Endoscopy is also a valuable diagnostic tool, enabling the veterinary clinician to directly identify regions of inflam- mation within the esophagus.

Following diagnosis, treatment of esophagitis is aimed at correcting any primary problems that may be present, reducing inflammation with anti-inflammatory drugs, preventing secondary infections with appropri- ate antibiotics, and reducing the amount of stomach acid secretions using medications designed for this purpose.

Hairballs

As far as elderly felines are con- cerned, hairballs are by far the most prevalent type of gastrointestinal foreign body seen. Caused by the accumulation of hair within the stomach and upper portion of the small intestine secondary to feline grooming activity, *hairballs* are the leading cause of sporadic vomiting in cats. As one might expect, the incidence of this problem increases during the spring and fall months during the normal shedding cycles.

In most cases, diagnosis of hairballs is relatively straightforward, as elongated masses of hair are usually expelled during vomiting episodes. However, in those instances in which the accumulation of hair has become so great as to prevent its expulsion out through the esophagus or transport through the intestines, diagnosis may become more difficult. In these cases, a combination of clinical signs exhibited, physical exam findings, and, if needed, radiographs of the abdomen can be helpful in confirming the cause. Direct examination of the stomach and upper small intestine using an endoscope can provide positive identification of hairballs and allow for their subsequent removal.

Standard treatment for cats that frequently accumulate hairballs in their digestive tract involves the daily administration of a commercially available hairball remedy or laxative paste to lubricate the hair mass and ease its passage. In the same way, recurrences can be minimized by the administration of the laxative one to two times a week on a routine basis.

Gastrointestinal Ulcers

Ulcers are caused by the loss or breakdown of the protective mucus barrier covering the inner surfaces

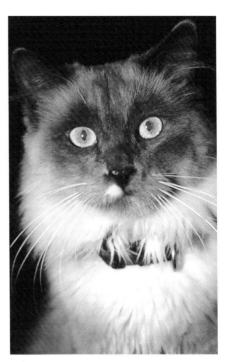

Hairballs are more common in those cats with medium to long hair coats.

of the digestive tract, allowing stomach acids, bile acids produced in the liver, or toxins to erode and digest the lining of the stomach and intestines. In aged felines, the most prevalent causes of ulcer formation is kidney disease, although neoplasia, stress associated with acute or chronic illness, foreign bodies, and prolonged therapy with certain types of drugs, such as anti-inflammatory agents can lead the ulcer formation. Symptoms exhibited by cats with digestive system ulcers can include loss of appetite, weakness, vomiting, and/or diarrhea. If the ulcerations are extensive, they may cause bleeding, which may manifest itself as black, tarry stools and/or blood-tinged vomitus.

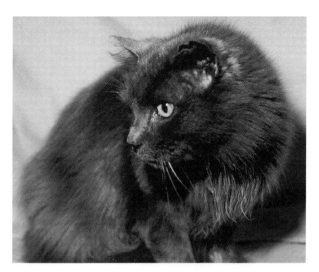

Diagnosis of eosinophilic enteritis is made through examination of biopsy samples taken from affected organs. Treatment consists of corticosteroids to reduce the inflammatory response. Relapses following therapy are common, necessitating long-term medical and dietary management.

Inflammatory Bowel Disease (IBD)

Inflammatory bowel disease (IBD) in cats is actually a group of chronic digestive disorders characterized by the infiltration of the walls of the bowels with inflammatory cells, leading to abnormal wall thickening and irregularities. Only in recent years has IBD been recognized as a significant cause of chronic vomiting and/or diarrhea in cats. As far as the cause of IBD is concerned, research to date has failed to uncover an exact cause. Many veterinarians believe that bacterial and/or dietary proteins may stimulate an autoimmune type of reaction in these cats. This reaction, in turn, manifests as a buildup of immune cells on and within the surfaces coming in contact with these proteins. Interestingly enough, it has also been noted that inflammatory bowel disease occurs simultaneously in over 35 percent of those older cats suffering from hyperthyroidism.

The classic clinical sign associated with IBD in cats is chronic vomiting. Often misdiagnosed as hairballs, vomiting induced by IBD usually occurs intermittently over

The classic clinical sign associated with IBD in cats is chronic vomiting.

Ulcers are diagnosed based upon clinical signs and physical exam findings, as well as radiography and endoscopy. Treatment efforts are geared toward correcting any underlying cause, and administering drugs designed to reduce stomach acid secretions or to replace the protective coatings over the ulcerated areas.

Eosinophilic Enteritis

Eosinophilic enteritis is a disease characterized by a thickening and inflammation of the walls of the intestinal tract caused by an infiltration of white blood cells. At the same time, this infiltration can enlarge and inflame other organs of the abdomen, including the liver, spleen, and lymph nodes. Clinical signs associated with this disorder include vomiting, diarrhea, and weight loss. The exact cause of this disorder remains unknown; however, allergies are believed to be involved.

months to years, gradually worsening and increasing in frequency with time. In addition to vomiting, bloody diarrhea and abdominal pain are also clinical signs seen in cats suffering from IBD.

Diagnosis of IBD in cats is made through the use of a thorough history, physical exam findings, radiographs of the abdomen, and, more specifically, biopsy samples from affected portions of bowel. Diagnostic techniques such as these will help differentiate this condition from other disorders that may cause similar clinical signs, including foreign bodies, hyperthyroidism, pancreatitis, lymphosarcoma, and bowel obstruction.

Treatment for inflammatory bowel disease in felines employs the use of drugs designed to reduce the inflammatory response, as well as medications designed to locally suppress the immune system response within the gut. Administration of these medications may be required long-term to control this disorder. Most treatment regimens for IBD also require dietary adjustments using rations that are hypoallergenic. Unfortunately, the overall prognosis for cats suffering from IBD is very guarded. Lymphosarcoma is not an uncommon sequela to severe cases of IBD that cannot be controlled through medical means.

Colitis

Colitis refers to the inflammation of the lining of the large intestine.

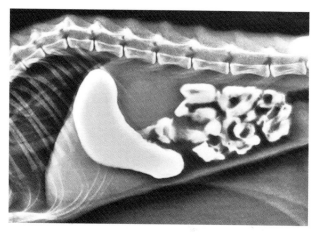

This inflammation normally results in a diarrheic condition that is characterized by an abundance of fresh blood and mucus in the stools. *Tenesmus*, or straining to defecate, is another clinical sign that may be seen in select cases of colitis due the irritation affecting the lower bowel.

Colitis in older cats falls under two categories: acute and chronic. *Acute colitis* refers to a sudden onset of symptoms that usually lasts only a few days with proper therapy. In contrast, *chronic colitis* is a long-term condition that may keep recurring over an entire lifetime, even with treatment. Acute bouts of colitis can occur secondary to such conditions as dietary indiscretions, viral and bacterial intestinal infections, parasites, foreign bodies, toxicities, and stress. Chronic colitis may result from diseases such as FeLV, FIV, autoimmune disorders, fungal infections, and tumors. Food allergies have also been implicated in

Contrast radiograph outlining the stomach and intestines of a cat with IBD.

several cases of chronic colitis in older cats that just didn't seem to clear up with conventional therapy.

Diagnosis of both acute and chronic colitis and their underlying causes is first approached using historical information, existing clinical signs, and physical examination. Stool examinations and other laboratory tests, especially feline leukemia and FIV testing (if not previously done), are essential in all cats experiencing colitis. Radiographs, including barium contrast studies, are indicated in select cases of chronic colitis. Colonic biopsies obtained surgically or through the use of an endoscope can also prove to be helpful for establishing a conclusive diagnosis of the underlying cause of the inflammation.

Treatment of colitis in older cats is geared toward the underlying cause. Any dehydration caused by the diarrhea must be corrected at once using intravenous fluids to correct the deficits. Parasites should be treated using proper dewormers and antiparasitic medications. Antibiotics can be used to help remove any disease-causing bacteria within the colon, and steroid anti-inflammatories may prove to be helpful in abating clinical signs associated with inflammation. If polyps or tumors are presented, surgery may be necessary to generate a cure. Unfortunately, many cases of chronic colitis, especially those caused by stress or by immune system disorders, cannot

be cured completely. In these cats, treatment goals are aimed at reducing the magnitude of the recurrences. Anti-inflammatories, antibiotics, and medications such as kaolin and pectin that coat and soothe the lining of the colon can help provide relief from these intermittent flare-ups.

Dietary management is an important factor in the treatment of colitis. Upon initial flare-ups, bland, easily digestible diets can help calm most irritated colons. As with people, chronic, recurring bouts of the disease can often be effectively managed by increasing the fiber content of the ration, which promotes normal and regular bowel movements. Lastly, if a food allergy is diagnosed, a hypoallergenic diet is the correct choice for colitis in cats.

Feline Megacolon

Feline megacolon is a disease condition characterized by fecal buildup and impaction within the colon due to the inability of the organ's muscular walls to contract and expel its contents properly. This disease condition in older cats is caused by a disruption in or absence of nervous activity within the colonic walls. Nervous interference may be caused by trauma to the spinal cord and/or nerves innervating the colon, or by other diseases affecting the nervous system.

The clinical signs associated with feline megacolon are related to the constipation it causes, and include frequent, painful attempts to defecate (the most obvious sign), vomiting, dehydration, loss of appetite, and abdominal pain. Diagnosis is based upon clinical signs, physical exam findings, and radiographic analysis of the abdomen, which usually reveals gross dilatation of the colon. Treatment of megacolon involves removing the fecal impaction using warm water enemas and by infusing the colon with mineral oil. Enemas designed for use in humans should not be used in cats, as the components contained within can cause severe dehydration in felines. Specific drugs, such as cisapride, may be prescribed to help stimulate motility within the diseased colon. Severe cases of megacolon may require patient sedation and manual evacuation of the bowel by a veterinarian. Supportive treatment in the form of intravenous fluids to combat dehydration and potassium supplements to fight hypokalemia may be needed in these instances as well.

Because a total cure for this condition is difficult to obtain, most cats with megacolon require consistent preventive maintenance therapy to minimize repeated flare-ups. Daily administration of oral hairball laxatives and stool softeners is indicated to keep bowel movements regular. Increasing the amount of fiber offered in the diet has also been shown to be helpful in preventing relapses. Finally, surgical procedures that entail the removal of diseased, weakened portions of the colon may be called upon as means of control for this troublesome condition.

Anal Sac Disease

The anal sacs are anatomical structures located beneath the skin on either side of the anal opening in cats. Their function is to produce a special fluid, quite odorous in nature, that serves as an identification marker for other cats. Although the contents of these sacs are normally expressed with bowel movements or urine spraying activity, many owners find, to their dismay, that their pet can also express these sacs at will when stressed or frightened!

Anal sac disease is relatively rare in older cats, yet it can occur. Inadequate emptying of the sac(s) may occur secondarily to allergies and other sources of skin inflammation, diarrhea, constipation, parasites (such as tapeworms), dietary changes, and, importantly in cats, obesity. Over time, the retained fluid within the sac(s) becomes thick and gritty, leading to impaction, and ultimately infection.

Signs associated with anal sac impaction and infection in cats include constant licking and grooming in the perineal region, localized pain and swelling, and in advanced infections, draining tracts of pus exiting from the skin surrounding the sacs. Diagnosis is made upon physical examination.

Impactions of the anal sacs are treated by the manual expression of the sacs. Infected anal sacs are first emptied in the same way, then instilled with antibiotic ointment. Oral antibiotics may also be used to expedite recovery. These procedures should only be performed by a qualified veterinarian. In some instances, sedation or anesthesia may be necessary if the discomfort is too great.

Anal sac disease in cats can usually be prevented through diet. Increasing dietary fiber will promote more frequent bowel movements and thus more frequent emptying of the sacs. In addition, encouraging weight loss in obese cats through dietary changes will also reduce the incidence of problems. Finally, for recurring bouts of anal sac infection, actual surgical removal of the anal sacs is a viable option to eliminate this problem once and for all.

Pancreatitis

The pancreas is an organ responsible for the production of essential digestive enzymes that break down foodstuffs into usable and absorbable units within the small intestine. It is also the site of production for the hormone insulin, which is vital for the conversion of sugar (glucose) to energy within the body.

Inflammation involving the pancreas is termed *pancreatitis*. In older cats, the cause of most cases of pancreatitis remain unknown. Some cases result from abdominal trauma, tumors, intestinal obstructions, infectious diseases such as FIP and toxoplasmosis, liver and gall bladder disease, and insecticidal poisoning. Signs of pancreatitis include weakness, loss of appetite, excessive salivation, vomiting, diarrhea, dehydration, and abdominal pain. In addition, repeated bouts of pancreatitis can damage the insulin-producing cells of the pancreas, resulting in clinical signs associated with diabetes mellitus. Another aftereffect of chronic pancreatitis in cats can be a condition known as *exocrine pancreatic insufficiency*. Characterized by the inability of the pancreas to produce proper amounts of pancreatic digestive enzymes, exocrine pancreatic insufficiency is accompanied by a marked increase in appetite (due to poor digestion of nutrients), chronic weight loss, and diarrhea. This loose stool often contains large amounts of fat, which may cause a greasy soiling of the hair coat in the hind end.

Pancreatitis is difficult to definitively diagnose in cats. Traditional elevations in levels of amylase and lipase, two pancreatic enzymes, are not seen as consistently in cats as it is in dogs with the disease. Radiography, ultrasonography, and endoscopy can be employed as alternate diagnostic methods, yet even the reliability of these can be inconsistent. In most instances, diagnosis is based upon clinical signs seen and by diagnostic testing methods to rule out other potential causes of these signs. If exocrine pancreatic insufficiency is suspected, specialized laboratory tests will need to be performed on a series of stool samples in order to positively identify the condition.

Cats experiencing only a mild bout of pancreatic inflammation will often recover upon all food and water being withheld for at least 24 hours. When treating severe cases of pancreatitis, it is imperative that all food, water, and even oral medications be discontinued for at least 48 hours. Intravenous fluids will be required as well to prevent dehydration during this time. Additionally, antibiotics, pain relievers, and medications designed to reduce pancreatic secretions are usually employed to prevent secondary complications. Certainly all underlying disease conditions contributing to the pancreatitis must be addressed as well.

Upon recovery, cats should be maintained on a dietary ration that is low in calories and easily digestible to reduce the workload placed on the pancreas. For those cats that are overweight, increasing exercise levels and promoting weight loss will reduce their susceptibility to subsequent flare-ups. Finally, cats experiencing exocrine pancreatic insufficiency due to chronic bouts with this disease will require enzyme supplementation to their diet to ensure that adequate digestion of foodstuffs takes place.

Feline Liver Disease

The liver serves many vital functions within the feline body. It aids in the digestion of food and stores up sugars to be used at a later date by the body for energy. This organ is the site of synthesis of protein and fat molecules and acts as a storage depot for vitamins as well. In addition, certain components necessary for the proper clotting of blood are produced here. Probably the one function that sets this remarkable organ apart from the others is the detoxification of metabolic by-products and potentially poisonous substances that are introduced into the body. Obviously, with such a wide variety of vital functions, any malfunction of this organ can have serious health consequences.

In the elderly cat, liver damage can occur secondarily to a number of different diseases and conditions. For instance, lymphosarcoma and other FeLV-related diseases can impart serious damage to the feline liver. Other tumors that may arise from the liver tissue itself or metastasis from elsewhere in the body can interfere with its normal functioning as well. Infectious diseases such as FIP and bacterial infections, and internal diseases such as diabetes mellitus, pancreatitis, autoimmune disease, and cardiomyopathy can all damage otherwise healthy liver tissue. Toxic substances that are consumed or produced as by-products of metabolism can also overwhelm and damage a liver if concentrations reach high enough levels. Cats in general are sensitive to many types of drugs, including aspirin and acetaminophen because their livers lack an important enzyme responsible for metabolizing these medications. As a result, even small amounts of these agents can cause significant damage to a cat's system. In addition, as liver function decreases with age, it may become less efficient at breaking down those medications used to treat other disease conditions in older cats. For this reason, the dosages of any medications given to elderly felines should be monitored closely by a veterinarian and adjusted as necessary.

There are four types of liver disease that can arise in elderly cats. The first, *acute hepatic necrosis*, is characterized by direct damage to and subsequent death of liver cells resulting from exposure to toxic substances, bacterial or viral infections, tumors, and oxygen deprivation, such as that seen with poor circulation caused by cardiomyopathy. A second condition that can occur is a *bile duct obstruction*. Bile ducts transport bile produced within the liver to the intestines, where it aids in digestion. Obstruction to this flow causes bile to back up within the liver, damaging healthy liver cells. The most common cause of bile duct obstruction in cats is a mass of some type, be it a tumor, abscess, or granuloma. Thirdly, *cholangitis/cholangiohepatitis* are terms that refer to inflammation of the bile ducts and surrounding liver tissue. Because the bile ducts empty into the intestine in close proximity to the pancreas, this condition is often associated with inflammation of this organ as well. Cholangitis/cholangiohepatitis can result from bacterial insult to the liver, or from damage caused by an overreactive immune system responding to some internal disease. The fourth type of liver disease is called *hepatic lipidosis*, characterized by an extensive infiltration of the liver by fatty tissue that causes pressure on healthy liver cells and interferes with their function. Obese cats that suddenly lose weight or those cats exposed to prolonged periods of starvation are predisposed to hepatic lipidosis. Hepatic lipidosis should be considered a threat to cats that develop loss of appetite for any reason. To make matters worse, this condition tends to be self-perpetuating; that is, as the fatty deposition worsens, the appetite becomes depressed even more. As a result, prompt nutritional support, including force-feeding through a tube inserted directly into the stomach, is a must for felines experiencing appetite loss caused by disease or stress.

Clinical signs associated with diseases of the liver include loss of appetite (often profound), vomiting, diarrhea, and fever. *Jaundice*, or *icterus*, is seen in advanced cases of liver disease. This clinical manifestation is caused by elevated levels of substances called bile pigments (produced in the liver) within the bloodstream and is hallmarked by a yellow discoloration of the skin, mucous membranes, and blood serum. Still another symptom indicating advanced liver disease is ascites, or fluid buildup within the abdominal cavity. This is due to increased resistance to blood flow through the liver, which forces fluid out of the blood vessels and into the abdomen. Finally, cats suffering from advanced liver disease can also experience delayed blood clotting, anemia, and seizures, the latter occurring as ammonia and other toxins accumulate in the bloodstream.

Diagnosis of feline liver disease is based upon clinical signs, physical exam findings, biochemical test results on blood samples, and special liver function tests. Radiography and ultrasonography can also prove to be quite helpful in the assessment of liver disease. For definitive answers, actual liver biopsies may be obtained and microscopically examined by the trained eye.

Therapy for cats suffering from liver disease is aimed at preventing further damage or deterioration from taking place, and encouraging the replacement of diseased liver tissue with healthy tissue. Fortunately, the liver has the capability for regeneration and self-healing if the underlying insult is properly addressed. Until such healing can take place, intravenous fluids are required for these felines to prevent dehydration and to reduce stress. In addition, complete nutritional support is a must for proper recovery to occur. Easily digestible, protein-restricted diets are ideal for a patient suffering from a liver disorder. Owners may be required to learn how to tube-feed their cat during the recovery process to ensure that proper nutritional support is being achieved. Antibiotics are also useful in cats with liver disease to prevent secondary infections and, for those cases exhibiting neurological signs caused by too much ammonia in the bloodstream, to reduce the number of ammonia-forming organisms in the digestive tract. Fluid buildup within the abdomen can usually be managed with drugs designed to stimulate urination and by a reduction in the amount of sodium in the diet.

The Integumentary System

The skin and hair coat of the cat function to protect the body from intrusion by foreign invaders or substances, to provide a sensory awareness of the surrounding environment, to act as a storage site for water and nutrients required by the body, and to help regulate body temperature. The sebaceous glands located within the skin secrete oils (sebum) onto the skin, lubricating and moisturizing the outer body surface and hair coat and inhibiting the growth of bacteria or fungi on the skin surface. In addition, special structures such as pads and retractable claws serve in locomotion and defense, and help reduce the stress placed on bones and joints.

Seasonal shedding ensures that the hair coat remains fresh and vibrant. Triggered by increases or decreases in daylight, peak shedding periods for cats occur during the spring and fall months. For those felines that spend the majority of their time indoors, shedding may become a year-round phenomenon. Interestingly enough, cats have the special ability to shed their hair at will when they feel stressed or threatened. This ancestral trait was specifically designed to leave a cat's enemy with nothing but a mouthful of hair if a serious confrontation ensued!

Hair color is dependent upon the amount of pigment present within the hairshaft. Large amounts of pigment result in black hair; hairs that lack pigment are white. Graying that may occur with aging results from the gradual loss of pigment within these hair shafts.

As cats grow older, alterations in normal skin anatomy and function occur with greater frequency, and can predispose to disease. In addition, the skin and hair coat become susceptible to the outward manifestations of internal diseases that may originate in other organ systems (see Table 20). As a result, the appearance and integrity of the skin and hair coat of older cats can provide valuable insight into the overall health and well-being of the pet.

Allergies and Feline Dermatologic Responses to Disease

Allergies are responsible for many cases of itchy skin and hair loss seen in older cats. An *allergy* is nothing more than an exaggerated immune response to a foreign substance within or on the surface of the body. They may develop at any age during a cat's life, with the severity of reaction varying with each individual. The types of skin disease or reactions that result from these allergic responses can be classified into three groups: feline miliary dermatitis, eosinophilic granuloma complex, and psychogenic alopecia.

Miliary dermatitis is a term that refers to a specific way in which feline skin responds to inflammation and/or irritation. A miliary reaction is characterized by the formation of tiny bumps and crusts that frequent the head, neck, and tail regions of the body. In extensive cases, the entire body may be involved. Furthermore, this miliary reaction in itself is quite itchy, and exacerbates scratching, rubbing, and licking of the affected skin.

Apart from allergies, miliary dermatitis can also be caused by ringworm infections, bacterial skin infections, adverse reactions to medications and drugs administered, and fatty acid deficiencies in the diet. Treatment for feline miliary dermatitis is aimed at correcting the underlying cause for the disorder. For those cases in which an under-

Table 20:
Dermatological Manifestations of
Internal Diseases in Older Cats

Disease Condition	Dermatologic Appearance
Internal parasites	Seborrhea; itching; poor wound healing
Diabetes mellitus	Fatty nodules on skin (xanthomas); friable skin; hair loss
Hyperthyroidism	Reddened ears; rough hair coat; excessive shedding; rapid nail growth
Hyperadrenocorticism	Thin, friable skin; pigment changes; hair loss
Allergic reaction	Localized or generalized swelling; reddened skin; itching
Autoimmune disease	Itching; reddened skin; blisters; ulcers; bruising; jaundice; crusts
Nutritional deficiencies	Itching; hair loss; infections; seborrhea; poor wound healing
Pancreatitis	Seborrhea; itching; hair loss
Neoplasia	Lumps; nodules; surface ulcerations; rough hair coat; friable skin
Toxicities	Thickened skin; ulcers; hair loss; reddened skin; blisters
Kidney disease	Hair loss; seborrhea; pitting of the skin when touched; ulcers
Bleeding disorders	Jaundice; darkened color to skin; bruising; ulcers
Liver disease	Jaundice; poor wound healing; friable skin; rough hair coat
FeLV and other infectious diseases	Ulcers; abscesses; seborrhea; poor wound healing; itching; skin masses

lying cause remains a mystery, treatment with steroid anti-inflammatory medications can provide temporary relief from the clinical signs. Antibiotics are used in those instances in which bacterial infections are suspected.

A second type of allergic skin presentation is termed *eosinophilic granuloma complex*. These skin reactions are characterized by the appearance of raised, ulcerated skin lesions with associated hair loss occurring at various locations around the body, especially the neck, lips, lower abdomen, hind legs, and perineum. Raised, well-demarcated reddened ulcers appearing on the lips of affected cats are called *indolent ulcers*. These ulcers tend to occur more frequently in female cats than in males. Most appear on the upper lip, and if not treated, can turn into cancerous lesions. *Linear granulomas* are eosinophilic granulomas that can occur anywhere on the body, but especially frequent the back portion of the hind legs, mouth, and footpads. These ulcerations are yellowish to pink in appearance, and, as the name implies, they tend to run in a straight line down the affected portion of skin. Like indolent ulcers, these lesions occur more frequently in females than in males. With both eosinophilic ulcers and linear granulomas, pain and itching do not appear to be significant factors. In contrast, eosinophilic plaques are types of eosinophilic granulomas that are associated with intense itching. These appear as well-demarcated, raised ulcers, often bright red in appearance, located on the abdomen and on the upper, inside portions of the back legs.

Diagnosis of eosinophilic granuloma complex in cats is made based upon clinical signs and on microscopic examination of cells or tissues obtained from the lesions. Like miliary dermatitis, treatment with steroid anti-inflammatory drugs can be used to temporarily bring the skin lesions under control while the underlying cause is being investigated. In extensive cases that don't respond to steroid anti-inflammatories or other medications, radiation therapy or cryotherapy can be used as an alternate treatment method.

Psychogenic alopecia is the name given to still a third type of skin disorder in cats that can be instigated by allergies. This condition involves continuous licking, chewing, and scratching by affected cats, which results in symmetrical patches of broken, stubbled hair. The abdomen and the perineum are most often affected. In addition, a classic "stripe" of hair down the back is often seen due to licking activity. Oftentimes, cats will do their licking and chewing at night or in some location in the house away from human scrutiny leaving their owners baffled as to the possible cause of their pets' hair loss.

Although allergies are an important cause of psychogenic alopecia, they aren't the only ones. Internal parasite infestations, FUS, musculoskeletal disorders, stress, and neuroses (especially in Siamese, Burmese, and Himalayan cats) have all been implicated as causes of this disorder.

Diagnosis of psychogenic alopecia is primarily based upon clinical signs seen. Therapy for this condition is similar to that for miliary dermatitis, namely steroid anti-inflammatory medications and identification/treatment of the underlying cause. In addition, behavior-modifying drugs can be used in select instances as needed.

The allergies that manifest themselves as miliary dermatitis, eosinophilic granulomas, or psychogenic alopecia are categorized into four main groups: inhalant allergies (atopy), flea allergies, food allergies, and contact allergies.

Inhalant allergies, also referred to as *atopic dermatitis*, can be a significant source of allergic skin disease in older cats. Grass and tree pollens, molds, dander, house dust, and hair are just some of the substances that can cause atopic dermatitis in cats. Signs of this type of allergy can include facial rubbing, incessant licking, and chewing all over the body with subsequent hair loss. Skin lesions indicative of miliary dermatitis or eosinophilic granuloma complex may be present as well.

Diagnosis of atopic dermatitis is based upon a history of clinical signs (seasonal versus nonseasonal), response to treatment, and/or allergy testing. This latter testing, called intradermal skin testing, involves actual injections of potential allergy-causing agents into the skin and observing for distinct circular skin reactions (wheals).

Atopy in older cats can be treated with topical shampoos and medications, steroid anti-inflammatory drugs, or hyposensitization injections (allergy shots). Traditionally, steroid anti-inflammatory drugs have proven most useful in the control of the clinical signs associated with inhalant allergies. However, they should be used with prudence, because long-term continuous use can have deleterious side effects. Hyposensitization injections, on the other hand, contain extracts of the substance(s) identified by intradermal testing as causing the atopy. By using a series of injections given at predetermined intervals, the body can often be conditioned to ignore the presence of the offending substance, thereby reducing the allergic response. Good success rates have been reported by some veterinarians using this method of therapy. However, results will vary depending upon geographic location, the particular veterinarian performing the testing and treatments, and the individual cat involved.

Next, *food allergy dermatitis* in older cats typically manifests itself as itching, hair loss, and skin lesions involving the face and neck regions, although any part of the body can be affected. Food allergies have even been implicated as one cause of recurring ear infections in cats. In addition, diarrhea, vomiting, and other digestive system maladies may occur with this type of allergy as well, often tipping off the astute veterinarian to a tentative diagnosis. An actual diagnosis of a food allergy is achieved through the use of food allergy trials in which the patient is fed a veterinary-available diet consisting exclusively of hypoallergenic protein source, such as lamb, turkey, or rabbit. If a positive response is seen within a six-week period, then the cat is placed back on its old diet. If clinical signs return, then a diagnosis of food allergy is made. Treatment consists of maintaining the cat on the hypoallergenic diet indefinitely to prevent recurrence of clinical signs.

A third category of allergic dermatitis in cats is the *flea allergy*. Apart from the itching and irritation caused by the mechanical action of fleas biting the skin, their saliva can also cause an allergic response, which makes the itching and hair loss even worse. The clinical signs associated with a flea allergy, which usually include a miliary response, tend to localize either on the head and neck, or along the back (especially near the base of the tail). Owners may fail to suspect fleas as the cause of their cat's itching and skin lesions simply because they fail to see any of the parasites on the skin. However, because cats are so efficient at grooming themselves and removing fleas, and because these parasites spend much of their time off of their host, fleas may not be located on the pet itself.

Diagnosis of a flea allergy is made based upon the clinical signs seen, and by the presence of fleas or their droppings on the cat's skin. In addition, the presence of tapeworm segments in the cat's stool or on the hair coat is highly indicative of a flea infestation, even though actual fleas may not be seen.

As one may expect, flea control is the treatment of choice for this disorder. In addition, steroid anti-inflammatory drugs can be used to provide temporary relief from the clinical signs until adequate flea control can be achieved.

Finally, *contact allergies* are immune responses by the body to irritating substances that may come in contact with the skin. Frequent offenders include detergents, shampoos, sprays, insecticides, flea collars, carpets, bedding, and plastic bowls used for feeding. Clinical signs seen consist of redness, itching, and swelling of the affected skin, especially at points of contact such as the face, abdomen, and/or feet. Diagnosis of a contact allergy is made from the type and location of clinical signs, and by separating the cat from the suspected offending agent and observing for a clinical improvement. Treatment is achieved by permanently removing the offending agent from the cat or environment. In the case of sprays, chemicals, or other topical agents causing the contact allergy, thorough rinsing of the skin and hair coat with water should be performed, followed by the administration of prescribed topical antibiotics or anti-inflammatory medications to fight existing clinical signs.

Seborrhea

Skin that is excessively flaky or oily is said to be seborrheic in nature. *Seborrhea* is caused by abnormalities in the production of keratin, which lines the outer surface of the skin and consists of dead epithelial cells. It is not considered a common primary disease entity in cats; however, due to internal changes associated with aging, older cats may be more prone to its development secondarily to various disease conditions. These can include allergies, nutritional deficiencies, skin parasites, and skin infections.

Seborrhea sicca is a type of seborrhea characterized by dry, flaky skin, hair loss, and itching. It often occurs secondary to external skin parasitism, low environmental humidities, fatty acid deficiencies, and poor grooming habits. A second presentation of seborrhea in cats, called *seborrhea oleosa*, consists of scaly, greasy skin and hair, occasionally accompanied by skin inflammation and hair loss. This type of seborrhea is seen with FeLV infections, liver disease, and autoimmune disease. A third type of seborrhea, *tail gland hyperplasia*, involves a collection of sebaceous glands located on the back near the base of the tail. This type of seborrhea is typified by an accumulation of yellow to black waxy debris that mats the hair coat in this region due to overactivity by these glands. Localized secondary bacterial infections are not uncommon in these cases as well. The exact cause of tail gland hyperplasia remains a mystery, yet poor grooming activity and hormonal influences have been implicated. A final type of seborrheic skin condition that may be seen in older cats is *feline acne*. This disease is characterized by the formation of blackheads and/or pustules on the chins of affected cats. Although the exact cause for this disorder remains unknown, many researchers feel that it is related to the cat's inability to adequately groom itself in this area. In addition, contact allergies may play a role in its development.

Diagnosis of seborrhea in older cats is based primarily upon type and location of clinical signs. Identification of the underlying cause is a must for effective treatment of secondary seborrhea. Treatment of seborrheic sicca involves the frequent use of gentle, nonallergenic shampoos and sprays to help moisturize the skin. For seborrhea oleosa, shampoos containing benzoyl peroxide or sulfur can be used to cut through the grease and soothe the skin. (Note: certain commercially available antiseborrhea shampoos containing salicylic acid or coal tars are toxic to cats and should not be used. Always read label precautions.) Unless otherwise directed by a veterinarian, medicated shampoos should be performed every three to four days for the first two weeks, then as needed on a weekly basis. Daily brushing should be performed on all cats with seborrhea. Finally, nutritional supplements and steroid anti-inflammatory medications have

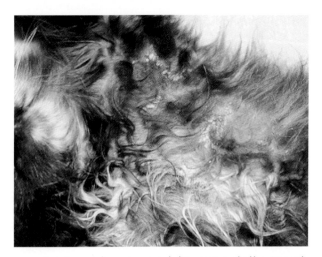

Superficial skin infection secondary to hair matting.

ance, FEA is primarily seen in those older cats that were neutered at a young age.

Diagnosis of FEA is based on ruling out other potential causes of hair loss, and upon experiencing a positive response to therapy. Treatment consists of sex hormone injections given at regular intervals. Side effects from such therapy are usually minimal when administered properly. In addition to sex hormones, thyroid hormone supplementation has also been used to stimulate hair regrowth in these cats.

Abscesses and Bacterial Skin Infections

Superficial bacterial skin disease can occur secondary to trauma, malnutrition, parasitism, hormonal abnormalities, and immune system malfunctions. Superficial infections appear as moist, raw regions with a thin covering of pus, or as crusts and scabs on the skin. In addition, if the hair follicles are infected (folliculitis), hair loss may be noted.

In contrast to superficial infections, *deep bacterial infections* involve the deepest layers of the skin and underlying tissues. Cellulitis and abscesses are two categories of deep infections that occur secondary to tissue injury, usually as a result of a bite wound from another cat. Sites most often affected include the face, extremities, and back near the base of the tail. Cellulitis refers to a poorly defined region of inflammation involving the skin and underlying tissue, whereas

been used in especially tough cases to alleviate clinical signs associated with these two types of seborrhea.

Treatment for tail gland hyperplasia and feline acne consists of clipping the hair away from the affected regions and scrubbing the site biweekly with an approved antiseborrheic shampoo, followed by a thorough drying of the region.

Feline Endocrine Alopecia (FEA)

Feline endocrine alopecia (FEA) is a condition resulting in a nonitchy, symmetrical hair loss affecting the abdomen, thighs, and perineum. Apart from this lack of itching, FEA can be further differentiated from allergy-induced psychogenic alopecia by an actual absence of hair in the affected regions, versus the broken and stubbled hair seen with the latter disease. Thought to be caused by a sex hormone deficiency or imbal-

abscesses have well-defined borders that distinguish them as distinct masses. Both can be characterized by a painful buildup of pus, and usually cause fever and depression.

Diagnosis of a bacterial infection is based upon the presence of pus or other clinical signs, such as crusts, scabs, and hair loss. Laboratory analysis of the blood will usually reveal an elevated white blood cell count in response to the foreign invaders. To further identify the causative organism and the antibiotics to which it is sensitive, bacterial cultures and sensitivity testings may be performed on discharges or crusts obtained from the skin and/or underlying tissues.

Most superficial skin infections can be treated using topical antibacterial creams, ointments, or drying agents for local infections, and medicated shampoos for those with more generalized distributions. In those cases in which remission cannot be achieved by the above means, antibiotics administered orally or by injection may be used. Both cellulitis and abscesses can lead to serious internal infections and blood toxicities if not treated in a timely manner with high doses of such antibiotics. Adjustments to the antibiotic being used should be made if culture/sensitivity occurs. Also, if well demarcated, abscesses can be lanced and flushed with medications to help speed recovery.

Ringworm (Dermatophytosis)
Ringworm is the most prevalent

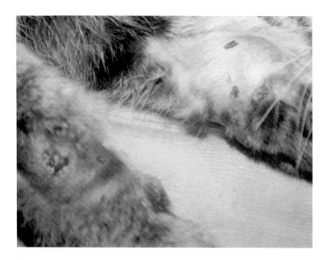

Cat bite abscesses.

fungal infection seen in cats. There are three different fungal agents that have the potential to cause ringworm in cats, the most common being *Microsporum canis*. Ringworm fungi invade the hair, nails, and superficial layers of the skin of infected cats. Living on dead tissue, these organisms produce allergic substances that cause hair loss and varying degrees of skin reactions. Interestingly enough, the organism is so well adapted to felines that many cats show no signs of infection whatsoever, and

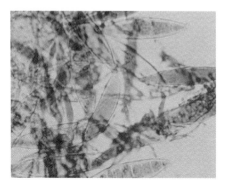

Ringworm fungal spores.

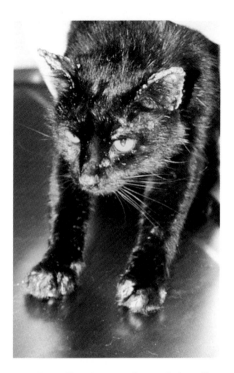

Older cat with a severe case of ringworm, coupled with mange.

present, it should become evident upon the fungal culture within five to seven days. Also, in cases where *Microsporum canis* is involved, evaluation of the affected skin and hair using a black light may reveal fluorescent pigments produced by the organism, thereby offering immediate identification. Although most cases of ringworm in cats are self-limiting (will clear up on their own without treatment), treatment should be instituted to prevent the spread of the disease to other cats and to people. This treatment includes shaving the affected areas to get rid of infected hairs, using medicated shampoos and topical antifungal medications to kill the remaining organisms, and, in especially extensive cases that fail to respond to topical treatments, orally administering the drug griseofulvin for a period of four to six week to accomplish the same.

can be effective carriers of the disease not only to other cats, but to people as well.

Transmission of ringworm can occur either through direct contact between cats or through contact with inanimate objects or soil that an infected cat may have rubbed against. Ringworm infections are characterized by patchy hair loss, often circular in nature, on the head and body. In addition, crusty inflamed skin, seborrhea, and pigmentation may be seen in response to infection. Diagnosis of this disease can be achieved by plucking hairs from a suspected region on the hair coat and then placing these hairs on a special fungal culture medium. If a ringworm infection is

Because ringworm contamination within an environment can persist for months, thorough disinfection of a cat's litter box and bedding should be performed to prevent reinfection. Also, by limiting interaction with stray animals and by screening new cats for ringworm prior to their introduction into a household, unexpected infections with these fungi can be avoided.

Sporotrichosis

Sporotrichosis is a fungal disease in cats caused by the soil-borne organism *Sporothrix schenckii*. After gaining entrance into the cat's body via puncture wounds from thorns (especially rose thorns), slivers, or scratch wounds, the fungal organism causes numerous disease-infected lumps and nodules, often ulcerated and draining, along the face, ears, neck, and legs. Rhinitis is another common manifestation of sporotrichosis in cats. Affected cats exhibit sneezing, nasal discharge, and facial swelling.

Diagnosis of sporotrichosis is based upon clinical signs and distribution of lesions, as well as microscopic examination of drainage and discharges. The treatment of choice for this fungal organism is sodium iodide. Because cats are ultrasensitive to this therapeutic agent, they must be monitored closely for signs of iodine toxicity throughout the duration of the treatment. Such signs can include weakness, vomiting, muscle tremors, hypothermia (low body temperature), and shock.

Like ringworm, sporotrichosis can cause disease in people and warrants respect whenever treating a cat so afflicted. As a result, gloves should be worn whenever handling or treating a cat with open, draining lesions in order to avoid accidental contamination with the organism.

The Immune System

The immune system consists of a complex interaction of specialized organs, cells, and chemicals, all

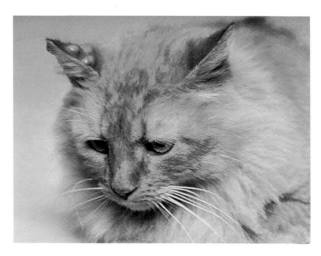

designed to protect the body from foreign invaders and neoplastic cells. Without it, a body would be quickly overcome and destroyed by a hostile environment. Although genetics plays the primary role in determining the strength and efficiency of this system, other factors, such as good nutrition, reduced stress, and priming with routine immunizations certainly contribute to the efficacy of the immune response.

Organs of the immune system include the bone marrow, thymus, spleen, and lymph tissue found throughout the body. The *bone marrow* is the origination site of the various immune system cells. The *thymus gland*, located at the base of the neck in young animals, plays an important role in the maturation of immune cells. It slowly regresses as a cat grows older. The *spleen* is an organ located within the abdomen. It acts as a filter and storehouse for blood and immune

Lumps on the surface of the ear caused by sporotrichosis.

cells. Finally, *lymphatic tissue* and glands found throughout the body help filter lymphatic fluid and blood of foreign matter.

Cells of the immune system include neutrophils, monocytes, macrophages, and lymphocytes. *Neutrophils* are white blood cells that engulf and destroy bacteria that gain entrance into the body. Assisting the neutrophils are *monocytes* and *macrophages*, immune cells that not only consume bacteria, but viruses, fungal organisms, and foreign matter as well. *Granulomas*, which are firm masses commonly mistaken for tumors, consist of conglomerations of macrophages and other cells that surround and imprison foreign matter, preventing its spread within the body. *Lymphocytes* are the immune cells responsible for producing antibodies against disease organisms and foreign tissues. These cells require periodic priming through immunization to ensure that they are ready at all times to produce protective levels of antibodies should an actual invasion occur. Certain types of lymphocytes are also responsible for destroying cancerous cells as they arise within the body.

Lastly, the immune system produces chemicals that aid in the stimulation and modulation of the immune response and in the destruction of foreign invaders and tumor cells. Included in these chemicals are interferon, interleukins, and complement. Much research is being devoted to the study of such chemicals and their effects in hopes of harnessing their power for concentrated use in the treatment against cancer and other devastating illnesses.

Allergic Reactions

Allergic reactions result from overblown responses by the immune system to foreign organisms or substances that have gained entrance into or have attached onto the body. These reactions can occur following the administration of medications or vaccinations, exposure to environmental irritants, insect bites and stings, or the ingestion of certain foods or poisons. The extent of the allergic reaction that takes place depends on the amount of previous exposure to the allergy-causing agent, and upon the extent of the current exposure.

Clinical signs seen with mild to moderate allergic reactions include intense itching, hives, soreness, vomiting, swelling, fever, and weakness. These signs may appear minutes to hours following exposure to the offending agent. On the contrary, life-threatening allergic reactions, known as *anaphylactic reactions*, can arise within seconds of exposure, and can cause breathing difficulties, collapse, shock, and even death. An allergy to bee or wasp venom is one example of an allergic response that can turn anaphylactic if prior exposure has taken place.

Allergic reactions are diagnosed by the clinical signs seen and the timeliness of their onset. Treatment for mild to moderate allergic reactions includes antihistamines to halt the further progression of the clinical signs, and steroid anti-inflammatory medications to reverse existing symptoms. In instances of anaphylactic shock, intravenous fluid therapy, large doses of antihistamines and steroids, and oxygen therapy are needed to counteract the effects of the reaction.

Autoimmune Disease

Like allergies, autoimmune diseases are caused by exaggerated responses by the body's immune system. However, instead of the reaction being directed toward some foreign substance or invader, an autoimmune response is mounted against the body's own tissues and organ systems. Owing to the immense power of the immune system, autoimmune diseases can devastate the health of an older cat.

Pemphigus complex is a series of autoimmune diseases that can cause severe ulcerations, crusts, and blisters on the skin of cats, especially around the mouth, lips, nose, and footpads. In addition, these lesions are often itchy and extremely painful. Because of the loss of skin integrity, secondary bacterial skin infections can complicate matters as well.

Systemic lupus erythematosis (SLE) is another autoimmune disease that can cause skin lesions similar to those seen with pemphi-

gus complex. In addition, this disease can cause damage to other tissues and organs within the body. Blood-clotting disorders, anemia, and kidney failure have all been linked to SLE in cats. Also, affected felines may experience painful arthritis as the immune system attacks the various joints of the body.

Autoimmune hemolytic anemia (AHA) is a condition in which perfectly healthy red blood cells are destroyed by the body in such numbers as to cause anemia. Cats suffering from AHA often experience extreme weakness and jaundice. *Immune-mediated thrombocytopenia* (IMT) involves a similar reaction by the body, but this time it is against the blood platelets. As a result, cats with IMT experience blood-clotting disorders that can be life threatening.

Finally, in rare instances, the body's immune reaction to an invading organism or foreign substance may lead to organ damage, especially the kidneys (see Kidney Disease and Kidney Failure, page 83). Such damage can occur secondary to the formation of immune complexes, which consist of antibodies

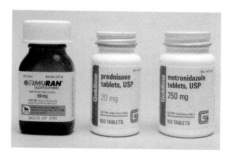

Medications commonly used to treat autoimmune disease.

bound to the foreign invader, within the organ tissue. Organ failure may occur if the condition is not recognized and treated in time.

Diagnosis of autoimmune disease is made through the evaluation of skin and organ biopsies, as well as specialized blood tests. Regardless of the type of autoimmune disease that is diagnosed, treatment utilizes extremely high dosages of corticosteroid hormones, which have a suppressive effect upon the immune system. In especially difficult cases, other drugs that modulate and suppress the immune system, such as azathioprine and gold salts, may also be used in conjunction with the steroid hormones to control the autoimmune reaction.

Immunosuppression

Interference with normal immune function can have serious health consequences. A suppressed immune system leaves the body susceptible to, among other things, invasion by infectious organisms and growth of neoplastic cells. A certain degree of immunosuppression can occur as a result of the aging process, hence the increased susceptibility of older cats to infectious diseases and cancer. In addition to the aging process itself, other important sources of immunosuppression in older cats include FeLV, FIV, chronic disease and stress, kidney failure, and bone marrow disorders. Endocrine disturbances such as Cushing's dis-

ease can also significantly reduce the effectiveness of the immune response. Finally, radiation and certain types of drugs, including steroid hormones and drugs used to treat cancer, can leave the feline body susceptible to a variety of diseases due to their immunosuppressive effects.

A state of immunosuppression may be detected through laboratory analysis of the blood and bone marrow. If possible, treatment of the underlying cause of the suppression should be instituted as soon as a diagnosis is made. Depending upon the cause of the immunosuppression, anabolic steroids and other drugs designed to boost the body's immune system may be prescribed as adjuncts to therapy.

The Eyes, Ears, and Nose

Sensory function enables a cat to react to and interact with its environment. The senses operate in coordination with other organ systems to optimize their efficiencies and to protect them from harm. Unfortunately, as aging takes its toll, overall sensory function may diminish, decreasing these efficiencies and impairing the elderly cat's ability to efficiently cope with its environment.

The Eyes

Being nighttime hunters, the eyes of the cat are designed to provide a higher degree of visual acuity than their canine cousins. The feline eye contains a number of unique adaptations, such as the slit-shaped design of the pupil to allow for exceptional dilation in dimly lit or dark conditions. In addition, the ability of the eye muscles to allow the eye to focus in on objects and to detect even the slightest of movements of potential prey is highly refined. Cats, like dogs, possess within their eyes those structures necessary to perceive their world in color. Whether they actually take advantage of their presence is still debatable.

The anatomy of the eye is indeed unique. A large portion of the outer surface of the eyeball is covered and surrounded by a special membrane, pink in appearance, called the *conjunctiva*. A *nictitating membrane*, or third eyelid, is also present at the inside corner of each eye. Designed to protect the eye during aggressive encounters, this lid will also often protrude over the surface of the globe with dehydration and/or disease. The clear, transparent membrane covering the front portion of the eye is called the *cornea*. As light passes through the cornea, it is directed through the pupil formed by the colored *iris*, which regulates the amount of light allowed into the eye. The *lens* of the eye is stationed just behind the iris. It serves to gather light and focus it on the *retina* lining the back wall of the eye. It is here that light is converted into nervous impulses. These impulses are then sent to the brain along large nerves, resulting in a perceived image. The *tapetum* is a layer of pigment that also lines the rear surface of the inner eye. It is a reflective device that improves night vision in cats and is responsible for the characteristic green glow seen when light is shone into the eyes of cats.

As with the other senses, aging takes its toll on vision as well. Reduced sensitivity of the nervous endings located within the eyes, combined with anatomical changes of other ocular structures, can result in diminished sight. In addition, several diseases that may interfere with vision can appear with greater frequency as a cat matures.

Glaucoma is a serious disease characterized by an increase in fluid pressure within one or both eyes. In older cats, glaucoma can develop secondary to a buildup of inflammatory material within the eye secondary to FIP or feline leukemia, luxation of the lens due to trauma or cataracts, tumor growth (lymphoma), and synechia, a term used to describe the iris "sticking" to the lens or cornea because of inflammation within the eye. Glaucomatous eyes appear reddened and inflamed, with blue, hazy corneas and dilated pupils. Blindness may also result from pressure damage to the retina. In severe cases, the affected eyeball may become noticeably enlarged and painful.

Diagnosis of glaucoma is confirmed with direct pressure readings

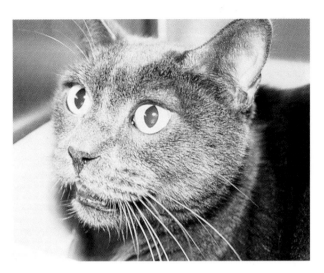

Cataract development in an elderly feline.

taken with a special instrument called a *tonometer*. Due to the destructive nature of this disease, prompt treatment is vital. Primary treatment goals are aimed at reducing the pressure within the eye as quickly as possible. Drugs designed to draw fluid out of the eye and back into the bloodstream will be initially used for this purpose. In addition, other medications that control the amount of fluid present within the eye will be used for long-term management. Anti-inflammatory drugs can also be employed to reduce the pain and inflammation associated with glaucoma. Once pain and pressure are brought under control, a diligent search for an underlying cause should be made if not yet identified. Once found, it should be treated accordingly. For example, chemotherapy employed to treat lymphoma within the eye will help prevent a repeat rise in eye pressure from occurring.

Also, in those instances in which a luxated lens is causing the increase in pressure, surgery may be necessary to remove the lens and correct the glaucoma. For those cases that fail to respond to medical or surgical therapy, removal of the affected eye may become necessary.

Cataracts and lenticular sclerosis: *Cataracts* are opacities of the lens that, in older cats, can develop secondary to such things as eye trauma, infections, or diabetes mellitus. The amount of visual impairment caused by the opacity is directly proportional to its maturity. In addition to mechanically obstructing vision, cataracts can also predispose the affected eyes to lens luxations and glaucoma.

True cataracts must be differentiated from another common condition seen in maturing cats, *lenticular sclerosis*. Caused by a hardening of the lens material, this condition differs from that of true cataracts in that light can still penetrate the discolored lens, thereby preserving visual function. Differentiation of the two conditions can be made by a trained veterinarian using a special instrument called an *ophthalmoscope*.

Treatment of cataracts involves surgical removal of the affected lens. This is accomplished by actually entering the eye and removing the lens intact or by using ultrasound to shatter the lens into smaller pieces, which are then extracted from the eye using specialized instruments inserted into the globe. Once the offending lens is removed, vision is usually restored. If desired, lens implants or replacements can also be utilized in cats to help sharpen vision even further.

Diseases of the retina: The *retina* is the structure within the eye that converts light impulses into nervous impulses that travel to the brain. With age, the efficiency and speed at which this function is carried out tends to decline somewhat, though usually not dramatically. However, if coupled with retinal insult caused by some other disease condition, significant visual impairment can arise.

A number of disease conditions can interfere with retinal function and cause partial or complete blindness. For instance, glaucoma affecting an eye can place so much pressure on the blood vessels supplying the retina of that eye that a secondary retinal degeneration results. Hemorrhages that blot the retinal surface may appear due to anemia or blood-clotting disorders. Retinal detachments and subsequent loss of function can occur secondary to FIP, toxoplasmosis, fungal infections, lymphosarcoma, kidney disease, poisonings, and trauma in elderly cats. Finally, nutritional deficiencies can lead to loss of retinal function as well. *Feline central retinal degeneration* is a condition characterized by the gradual degeneration of the retinas and sight in both eyes due to a deficiency of taurine in the diet.

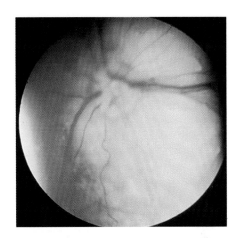

The retina of the eye as viewed through an ophthalmoscope.

Seen primarily in cats fed poor quality cat foods or table scraps, feline central retinal degeneration usually accompanies cardiomyopathy, also caused by taurine deficiency.

Diagnosis of retinal disease and its underlying cause is made using history, physical exam findings, laboratory blood tests, and information obtained from an ophthalmic examination of the retinas themselves. In addition, an *electroretinogram*, which measures the electrical activity taking place within the retinas, will provide a conclusive diagnosis of retinal-related blindness.

Fortunately, most cases of retinal disease in older cats tend to respond favorably to treatment if instituted properly and promptly. Retinal detachments will usually resolve on their own once the underlying problem has been treated. In addition, if started soon enough, taurine supplementation in the diet of deficient cats will usually reverse the changes that had taken place within the retinas. Finally, relieving the pressure placed on a retina by glaucoma should effectively restore sight in the affected eye(s), again, assuming timely therapy.

Corneal ulcers and scratches: Because of their role in gathering light and directing it to the lens of the eye, healthy corneas are essential for proper vision. Any inflammation involving these structures can seriously threaten eyesight if not managed promptly.

Important causes of corneal scratches, which may progress into a full-blown surface ulceration, can include trauma inflicted by a claw from another cat, foreign matter in the eyes, and other types of direct trauma to the corneal surface, such as accidental contact with shampoo or soap.

Symptoms of corneal surface injury include squinting, photophobia (avoidance of light), ocular discharge, and pain, exemplified by pawing at or rubbing the affected eye. A change in the normal color or transparency of the corneal surface is also an indicator of inflammation. Definitive diagnosis of a corneal lesion is achieved through the use of a special stain applied to the surface of the cornea.

If treated quickly and aggressively, corneal lesions usually heal quite rapidly. For ulcers involving only the superficial layers of the cornea, topical antibiotic ointments or solutions designed for use in the eyes and applied three to six times daily will help speed healing. Atropine drops or solutions designed to dilate the pupil to prevent painful spasms are also used to reduce the discomfort associated with the ulceration. In addition, dilating the pupil of the affected eye will also prevent adhesions from forming between the iris and the lens or cornea due to inflammation.

Deeper corneal ulcerations are treated the same way that superficial ulcerations are, yet require close observation for progression or worsening of the ulcer. Bacterial cultures of such ulcers are indicated to be certain that the antibiotics being used are effective against the organisms involved, if any. For deep ulcers that worsen, or even fail to respond to conventional treatment, surgical procedures designed to protect and strengthen the diseased portion may be necessary to speed healing or to prevent the cornea from experiencing a rupture.

Conjunctivitis and uveitis: *Conjunctivitis*, or inflammation of the conjunctival membrane of the eye,

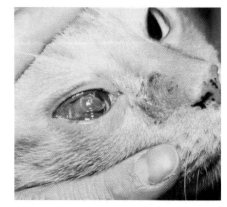

Green fluorescein staining of the surface of the eye revealing a corneal ulcer.

is the most common cause of "red eye" in cats. Clinical signs associated with conjunctivitis include a discharge, redness, swelling, and pain associated with the affected eye. Common causes of this condition include trauma (scratches), allergies, viral infections, bacterial infections, and foreign matter in the eye. The type of discharge present with conjunctivitis can often reveal the underlying cause (see Clinical Signs and Complaints, Discharge: Eye, page 162). Another cause of eye redness and pain in cats is termed uveitis. *Uveitis* refers to inflammation involving the inner portions of the eye, including the iris. Flare-ups of uveitis can be considered more serious than those associated with conjunctivitis, simply due to its location. Clinical signs associated with uveitis are the same as those for conjunctivitis, with the addition of iris discoloration, constriction of the pupil, and partial to complete blindness. Instigators of uveitis in elderly felines can be numerous. They can include trauma, FeLV, FIP, toxoplasmosis, bacterial and fungal infections, allergies, toxins, and neoplasia.

Because conjunctivitis and uveitis occur secondary to other problems, diagnostic tests performed will be directed at identifying the underlying cause. Careful ophthalmoscopic examination of the affected eye(s), with or without laboratory blood tests, will usually reveal a diagnosis. Corneal staining

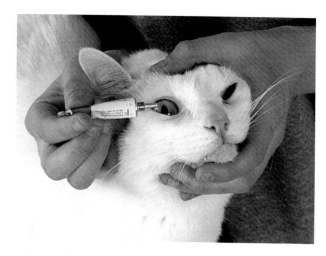

Conjunctivitis being treated with medicated ophthalmic ointment.

using a fluorescent stain is usually performed to determine whether or not the cornea is ulcerated.

Treatment of conjunctivitis is aimed at treating or eliminating any inciting causes, and at controlling the localized inflammation. If foreign matter is believed to be the source of the inflammation, thorough flushing of the eyes with a sterile saline solution on a daily basis for three to five days will help reduce the irritation. Medicated ophthalmic drops or ointments are indicated if a bacterial infection is present. In addition, ophthalmic preparations containing steroid anti-inflammatory medications can be useful in reducing inflammation and pain in those instances in which the corneal surface has not been damaged.

Cases of uveitis must be treated much more aggressively than conjunctivitis to prevent permanent damage to the interior of the eye. Strong doses of anti-inflammatory medications applied to the surface of the eye and given to the cat by oral or injectable means are indicated in these cases to bring them under control. If an infection is present, high doses of antimicrobial medications are indicated as well. Finally, special solutions or ointments designed to dilate the pupil are indicated as well to prevent adhesions from forming within the inflamed eye.

The Nose

The nose of the cat is designed for two basic functions. The first is to filter and warm inspired air prior to it entering the respiratory system. Special folds within the nasal cavity, called *turbinates*, can trap foreign debris and are rich in blood vessels that warm the inspired air. The second, and most obvious functions of the feline nose is olfaction, or smell. Air passing through the nose stimulates special hairlike receptors located at the top of the nasal cavities. Nerve fibers connected to these receptors then carry the signal generated to that portion of the brain responsible for perceiving and recognizing odors.

The sense of smell in cats, like dogs, is incredibly acute and precise, enabling them to detect even the most minute scents in their surroundings. In addition to its importance in the identification of people, animals, locations, and inanimate objects within the cat's environment, the sense of smell also exerts a strong influence on appetite as well. In fact, older cats that lose their sense of smell for whatever reason may refuse to eat, and become subject to the development of serious health consequences, such as hepatic lipidosis (see Feline Liver Disease, page 119).

Loss of smell: With advancing age, the nerve endings within the nose responsible for smell may slowly lose their sensitivity. This can also occur due to mechanical trauma to the nose, or upon exposure of the sensory endings to chronic infections, toxins, and irritants found in the air.

As the sense of smell diminishes, reduced appetites and behavioral changes often follow. Diagnosis of an olfactory (smell) disorder is accomplished through the use of special smell tests, and through examination of the nasal passages using an endoscope or radiographic procedures.

Unfortunately, there is no specific treatment that will restore olfactory sensitivity in older cats once it is lost. In an attempt to boost appetite, rations with strong aromas should be fed to help compensate for the sensory deficit. In addition, heating food prior to serving will help to increase its aroma. Cats with olfactory deficits should not be allowed to roam outdoors, because their ability to sense danger via their nose is compromised.

The Ears

The upper range of feline hearing is thought to exceed 60,000 cycles per second, close to three times the range of that for people. High pitches undetectable to the human ear can elicit a response from a cat, often to the bafflement of its owner. However, as with the sense of smell, the hearing capacity of cats diminishes with age as the nerve endings responsible for this function begin to wear out. In addition, various diseases and disorders can worsen hearing loss in older cats.

The feline ear consists of three sections. The first is the *external ear canal*, which communicates directly with the outside environment. Surrounding the opening of the external ear canal is the *earflap*, or *pinna*. In cats, the pinnae stand erect, supported by a strong band of cartilage. This feature allows for excellent air circulation within the external ear canal, a factor that helps explain why naturally occurring bacterial and yeast infections occur with less frequency in cats than in their floppy-eared canine cousins. Next, the *middle ear*, which is separated from the external ear canal by the *tympanic membrane*, or *eardrum*, acts as the bridge between this portion and the final section, the inner ear. The *inner ear* is the region that contains the special anatomical structures and nerve endings responsible for the sense of hearing. Disorders affecting any one of these three regions can be responsible for partial or complete deafness in older cats.

Ear infections: The external ear canal is separated from the middle ear by the tympanic membrane, or eardrum. In cats, this external portion of the ear can become infected with bacteria, fungi (yeast), and/or parasites. Clinical signs associated with an external ear infection include head shaking, itching, pain, and often an odorous discharge from the affected ears. Discharges from the external canal may become so profuse that hearing is adversely affected. Yellow to green discharges usually signify bacterial involvement, whereas brownish discharges are usually seen with yeast infections. Mixed infections are not uncommon as well. In the case of ear mites, a characteristic dry, black, flaky discharge will give away their presence.

Diagnosis of the causative agent can be made with a microscopic examination of the discharge. The type of treatment prescribed will depend upon the extent of the infection and upon the organism involved. Antibiotics and antifungal medications instilled directly into the external ear canal will help clear up most infections. Ear mite infestations may be managed with antiparasitic medications (see External Parasite Control, page 23). Also, because ear infections can occur secondary to other disease conditions such as skin allergies, identification and treatment of all underlying causes are essential for treatment success.

Like the external ear canal, the middle ear can become infected and inflamed, leading to hearing loss. Infections involving the middle ear usually result from long-standing infections of the external ear canal that penetrate the eardrum. The classic clinical sign associated with a middle ear infection is a noticeable head tilt to the side of the affected ear. In addition, because nerves supplying the muscles of the face pass through the middle ear, paralysis of these muscles, and a subsequent drooping of the eyelids, cheeks, and lips may occur secondarily to middle ear infections.

Diagnosis of a middle ear infection is confirmed by radiographing the suspected ear. Treatment consists of high doses of antimicrobial drugs to combat the infection, and anti-inflammatory medications to alleviate clinical signs. In severe cases, surgical drainage and medicated flushing of the middle ear canal may be needed to initiate healing.

Finally, because of direct communication with the middle ear, inner ear functions can also be disrupted by infections of the former. Additional signs that may be seen with inner ear infections include a loss of equilibrium, nausea, circling behavior, and an abnormal twitching of the eyeballs, called *nystagmus*. Also, because the nerve endings responsible for hearing are located in the inner ear, cats with untreated inner ear infections are at risk of developing nerve deafness. Diagnosis and treatment of inner ear infections are essentially the same as that for the middle ear.

Nerve deafness: Infections are not the only source of deafness in older cats. Nerve deafness can be inherited in some cats. This type of genetically induced deafness is seen primarily in white cats with blue eyes. In addition, age-related degeneration of the auditory (hearing-related) nerve endings can result in diminished hearing in elderly felines. Nerve deafness can also arise secondarily to trauma to the ear, toxins, or treatment of the ears with certain types of medications. For instance, certain types of antibiotics, called *aminoglycosides*, may be prescribed in older cats to combat certain types of bacterial infections. However, this class of drug can damage auditory nerves when used in high doses for extended periods of time. If this occurs, the damage is usually irreversible. As a result, veterinarians are especially cautious when selecting dosages and treatment durations of these and other drugs that may have similar effects upon hearing.

Diagnosis of nerve deafness is based upon history and special hearing tests. One such test, the *brain stem auditory evoked response test* (BAER), measures the brain's response to auditory stimuli and is quite helpful in the detection of hearing defects, determining the extent of any defect, and pinpointing its location. Unfortunately, no known treatment exists for nerve deafness once it is diagnosed. Most deaf cats will adapt to their condition with time. However, due to inherent dangers associated with environmental hazards, deaf cats should not be allowed outdoors unless closely supervised or maintained on a leash and harness.

Cancer in Older Cats

The term *neoplasia* refers to the uncontrolled, progressive proliferation of cells within the body. Bypassing the body's normal mechanisms for controlling growth, neoplastic cells reproduce at abnormal rates, often coalescing into firm, distinct masses called *tumors*. Neoplasia can be classified as either benign or malignant, depending upon the behavior of the cells involved.

Benign tumors consist of well-differentiated cells that divide and reproduce only slightly more rapidly than their normal counterparts. Such tumors are slow growing, well defined, and non-invasive, rarely spreading to other parts of the body. They seldom pose a threat to life unless their sheer size interferes with the function of an adjacent organ or, as in the case of glandular tumors, their presence alters the production of vital hormones.

On the contrary, *malignant* (cancerous) *tumors* experience frenzied growth, with uncontrolled spread (metastasis) to other organ systems within the body. In addition, these malignancies tend to spread with fingerlike projections far into the surrounding tissues (hence, the name "cancer"), making complete surgical removal next to impossible. Growth and duplication of these malignant cells continues until the cancer kills the cat or until every malignant cell is removed or destroyed. Death from cancer occurs when vital organs and tissues are replaced or starved to death by the malignant cells.

Tumors are further classified based upon their microscopic appearance and the body sites from which they originate. To identify benign tumors, the suffix "–oma" is used. For example, a benign tumor affecting bone would be referred to as an "osteoma," and one affecting glandular (adenoid) tissue would be called an "adenoma." On the other hand, malignancies involving epithelial or glandular cells end with the word "carcinoma," whereas those malignancies originating from any of

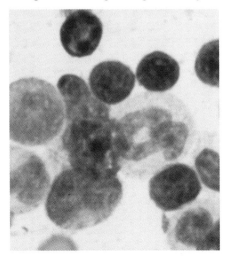

Neoplastic lymphocytes (small, dark purple cells) in a feline blood smear.

the remaining tissues of the body end with "sarcoma." For example, if the benign tumors referred to above were in fact malignant, the correct terms to use would be "osteosarcoma" and "adenocarcinoma" respectively.

Both carcinomas and sarcomas metastasize through the blood, with special affinity for the liver and lungs. Carcinomas also can spread via the lymphatic system, seeding lymph nodes with cancer cells along the way.

The effect that the aging process has on the development of neoplasia is still not fully understood. One current theory is that as cells continue to replicate throughout life, the chances of genetic mutations or accidents resulting from one of the replications increases due to the law of averages. Also, aging may impair the body's ability to combat cancer-causing viruses such as FeLV or to counteract the effects of *carcinogens*, substances or agents known to induce genetic mutation in otherwise healthy cells. Examples of carcinogens include ultraviolet radiation from the sun, airborne hydrocarbons, certain drugs and medications, and thousands of other chemicals that may be applied to the skin or ingested by cats.

Nonspecific clinical signs seen with neoplastic disorders are listed in Table 21. Neoplasia must be differentiated from abscesses, granulomas, and fungal diseases, all of which can be mistaken for tumors. Extreme care must be taken when determining whether or not a true neoplasia exists, because inflammation and secondary infection often accompany tumors, and can confuse the interpretation of test results.

Several methods and techniques are available to assist in the diagnosis of cancer in older cats. Diagnostic tests begin with a thorough history, evaluation of clinical signs, and a physical examination. Tumors affecting the skin, oral cavity, and other mucous membranes can usually be readily detected upon careful physical inspection. In addition, tumors residing within the abdominal cavity can often be detected by skilled palpation of the abdomen. Next, blood testing for the feline leukemia virus should always be performed on all cats suspected of having tumors, owing to the prevalence of this disease agent in the cat

Table 21:
General Signs
Associated with Neoplasia
in Older Cats

- Unexplained, pronounced weight loss
- Loss of appetite
- Chronic lethargy
- Firm, expanding lumps or masses
- Eating difficulties
- Breathing difficulties
- Persistent discharges
- Lameness
- Changes in urinary or bowel habits

population and its ability to induce neoplastic changes. Endoscopy, radiography, ultrasonography, and/or cytology are additional diagnostic tools used by veterinary practitioners to discover and identify neoplasia in cats. One benefit that endoscopy has to offer over the other techniques mentioned is that if a tumor is encountered, a biopsy of the neoplastic tissue can be immediately obtained through the instrument. A biopsy is by far the most reliable method of positively diagnosing neoplasia in cats. In fact, biopsies obtained from tumors and surrounding lymph nodes are often the only reliable resources used to determine whether a tumor is benign or malignant, and whether or not metastasis has taken place. Laboratory evaluation of the cells in the blood, serum biochemistries, urine, and in some instances, the bone marrow, may also assist in the detection of neoplasia that might not otherwise be apparent using other testing methods.

The type(s) of therapy chosen to treat a particular neoplasia is based upon six factors:

1. The type and characteristics of the neoplasm involved
2. The stage of its development, including the presence or absence of metastasis
3. The extent of spread and secondary organ involved if indeed metastasis has occurred
4. The cat's overall physical condition, including any preexisting medical disorders
5. Prognosis for remission or cure
6. Financial and quality of life considerations

Treatment options for neoplasms include surgery, radiation therapy, chemotherapy, cryotherapy, hyperthermia, and immunotherapy. Although other forms of therapy do exist, such as phototherapy and antiplatelet therapy, their use in veterinary medicine is limited. A combination of surgery, radiation, and chemotherapy is currently the most favored protocol for treating especially difficult malignancies in cats. As one may expect, the earlier a cancer is detected, the greater are the chances for complete cure.

Surgery is by far the most common method of treating neoplasia. As a rule, "if it is removable, remove it." In most instances, if a primary tumor that has not metastasized can be surgically removed along with a margin of healthy tissue surrounding the mass (as a safety precaution), a complete cure can be achieved with the surgery alone. Confirmation of complete removal can usually be verified through biopsy. Surgery is also useful for partial removal of tumors that for whatever reason cannot be fully removed. By decreasing the size of the tumor, temporary relief from clinical signs associated with the tumor can be achieved and the effectiveness of alternate treatments such as radiation therapy and chemotherapy can be improved. Finally, in extreme cases, surgical amputation of a limb may be required to eliminate a cancer. For example, osteosarcoma of bone is such an aggressive form of cancer that, in almost all cases, amputation of the affected limb is the treatment of choice.

Next, *radiation therapy* utilizes ionizing radiation to kill malignant neoplasms. Radiation is administered to feline patients over a two- to three-week period either through the use of an externally produced radiation beam or by radioactive implant. It exerts its effect by destroying the genetic material within the cancer cells, eliminating their ability to multiply. As a rule, radiation therapy is limited to those tumors with definable margins and ones that are slow to metastasize. As an adjunct to surgery, radiation therapy can be used to eliminate any microscopic neoplastic residues that may have been unknowingly left behind by the surgeon. Tumors affecting the bone marrow, skin, and digestive tract seem to be the most sensitive to this type of therapy.

A third mode of treatment, *chemotherapy*, involves the use of specific drugs designed to destroy neoplastic cells. Chemotherapy works on the premise that cancer cells are more sensitive to these chemical agents than are normal cells. This type of therapy is generally employed against tumors of the blood and lymph, and against those tumors that have metastasized (or are suspected of doing so), cannot be totally removed surgically, or are resistant to other forms of treatment. Some chemotherapeutic drugs commonly utilized in veterinary medicine include cyclophosphamide, vincristine, cytosine arabinoside, doxorubicin, L-asparagine, and prednisone. The efficacy of chemotherapy is generally increased by using combinations of these chemotherapeutic drugs rather than just one alone. This is due to the fact that each drug tends to exert a unique effect against the cancer cell; therefore, the neoplasia is attacked from multiple "directions" instead of just one. Furthermore, combining drugs will also increase the safety of the therapy, because it allows for the dosage of each drug to be lowered while still maintaining treatment effectiveness.

Side effects of chemotherapy in cats can include severe bone marrow depression, nausea, vomiting, and bleeding tendencies. Hair loss is rarely the problem in cats as it is in people. Fortunately, these side effects are dependent upon the doses of chemotherapy administered; hence, they can usually be controlled with proper adjustments to the dosage.

Freezing a tumor, or *cryotherapy*, is especially useful in treating masses involving the eyelids, mouth, and other areas where conventional surgery would be difficult to perform. With cryotherapy, tumors are rapidly frozen down to −20 degrees Celsius using liquid nitrogen, then slowly thawed. This cycle is repeated two to three times, depending upon the type of tumor involved. Following such treatment, death and regression of the mass usually result.

Hyperthermia is the just the opposite of cryotherapy. Hyperthermic therapy involves applying a source of intense heat to a localized neoplastic site in order to kill the neoplastic cells directly or disrupt the blood supply to them. Temperatures of up to 110°F (43°C) are used to accomplish the task. This type of therapy has been used with some success as the solitary means of treating select cases of feline squamous cell carcinomas; however, for most neoplasms, hyperthermia should be used in combination with other treatment methods in order to achieve the most favorable results.

Finally, a newer form of cancer therapy, *immunotherapy*, works to stimulate and support the body's immune system in its fight against the disease. In theory, by injecting immune-stimulating medications into the body, the resulting immune response will exact its revenge on neoplastic cells. In actual practice, much research and refinement is still needed to achieve these theoretical results. However, one form of passive immunotherapy that shows great promise in the treatment of cancer utilizes monoclonal antibody technology. Monoclonal antibodies are immune proteins that have been artificially cultivated within the laboratory. Highly concentrated preparations of monoclonal antibodies are being used to attack specific cancer cells directly and to carry chemotherapeutic drugs directly to the cancer cells, thereby increasing their effectiveness. Once refined, this technology should revolutionize the way in which certain cancers are treated, both in cats and in human beings.

For those cases in which prognostic or financial considerations may discourage treatment or call for its discontinuation, supportive measures may be instituted to improve the quality of life of a cat for the remaining days or weeks of its life. Surgical removal of cumbersome masses, antibiotic therapy to control secondary bacterial infections, and anti-inflammatory drugs to alleviate pain and discomfort are all palliative treatments that can be used in the terminal cancer patient. Of course, cats experiencing a rapid decline in quality of life or intense pain due to cancer growth should be considered for humane euthanasia to eliminate their suffering.

Select Types of Neoplasia in Older Cats

Because of the number of different types of organs and tissues within the body, there are a multitude of types of neoplasms that can arise in elderly cats. There are, however, certain types that appear more regularly than others.

Malignant lymphoma/lymphosarcoma (LSA) is by far, the most prevalent form of neoplasia encountered in older cats. This type of neoplasia, which is usually seen with a concurrent FeLV infection,

Table 22:
Top Five Tumors Arising in Older Cats

- Lymphoma/lymphosarcoma
- Leukemia
- Basal cell tumor
- Adenocarcinoma
- Squamous cell carcinoma

involves the neoplastic proliferation of white blood cells called *lymphocytes* within lymph nodes and lymphatic tissue throughout the body. There are a number of different presentations or forms of this particular neoplastic condition. *Alimentary* LSA primarily affects the intestines and associated lymphatic tissue. Other organs within the abdomen can be affected as well. Symptoms commonly seen with alimentary LSA include loss of appetite, weight loss, vomiting, diarrhea, bloody stool,

Swollen lymph nodes in the neck of an elderly cat suffering from LSA.

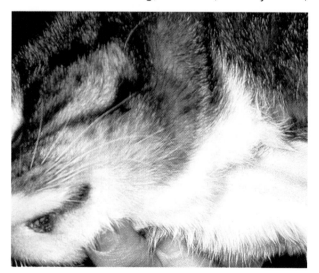

jaundice, and/or constipation. The mediastinal form of LSA presents itself as the proliferation of a large tumor within the chest cavity. Prominent signs include breathing difficulties, coughing, pleural effusions, chest wall incompressibility, and swallowing difficulties. *Multicentric* LSA affects lymph nodes and tissue in multiple sites throughout the body, all at one time. The signs seen with this type are variable, depending upon the organs most heavily involved. Prominent swelling of the lymph nodes, including those situated beneath the skin, is usually seen with this form of LSA. *Atypical* LSA is the name given to LSA that limits itself to solitary organs or organ systems within the body. Such solitary sites may include the skin, eyes, spinal cord, muscles, brain and kidneys, with symptoms reflecting the organ(s) involved. Finally, *lymphocytic leukemia* is a type of LSA characterized by the growth and proliferation of neoplastic lymphocytes within the blood and bone marrow, often affecting secondary structures such as the spleen and liver. Symptoms associated with lymphocytic leukemia tend to be nonspecific in nature, and can include anemia, jaundice, loss of appetite, weakness, fever, and organomegally (enlargement of internal organs).

Diagnosis of LSA can be achieved through cytology and biopsy of lymph nodes and suspect organs, radiographs of the abdomen and chest, and ultrasonography of the same. FeLV testing of these cats will often yield positive results, although not always. Treatment for malignant lymphoma involves chemotherapy, and in select cases, immunotherapy. Unfortunately, the prognosis a long-term remission (extending beyond six months) is poor for most affected felines.

Myeloproliferative disorders and leukemia are a family of disorders characterized by a neoplastic proliferation of the cellular components of the bone marrow, including the white blood cells, red blood cells, and platelets. Again, the feline leukemia virus is the culprit responsible for most myeloproliferative disorders seen in elderly felines. Symptoms associated with these disorders are often related to anemia and blood-clotting disorders (weakness, labored breathing, pale mucous membranes, loss of appetite), as the proliferating cells, especially white blood cells, within the bone marrow interfere with the normal production of red blood cells and platelets. In addition, certain myeloproliferative disorders are characterized by the abnormal production of the red blood cells and platelets themselves, leading again to those signs mentioned previously, and also to an enlargement of the spleen and liver. Definitive diagnosis of a myeloproliferative disorder is made upon the evaluation of the blood and a biopsy sample of the bone marrow. Unfortunately, because bone marrow transplants are not readily per-

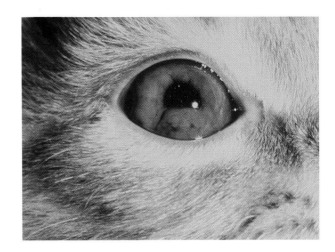

LSA involving the eye of a cat.

formed on cats, the overall prognosis for affected individuals is poor.

Basal cell tumors are the most common skin tumors seen in cats. These tumors, which are usually benign in nature, present as a firm, raised nodule with or without an ulcerated surface. They may also be heavily pigmented, appearing brown to black in color. Basal cell tumors originate from the deeper layers of the skin, hair follicles, and/or sebaceous glands. Sites most often affected include the skin of the head, neck, ears, and shoulder regions. These tumors can usually be treated quite successfully with surgical removal of the tumor, cryotherapy, or radiation therapy.

Mammary adenocarcinomas, another class of tumors that frequently affect older cats, form in response to extensive hormonal influences on mammary tissue, namely the hormone progesterone. Because progesterone is primarily a female sex hormone, these tumors are more likely to develop in females than in males.

These neoplasms can arise from a number of cell types within the mammary tissue itself, and can be benign or malignant in nature. Malignant mammary neoplasms grow quite rapidly, and tend to invade and cause inflammation in and around surrounding tissue. Metastasis to other organs such as the lungs, liver, bone, and kidney can occur as well. Mammary tumors in cats appear as hardened, sometimes painful swellings usually involving the forward-most glands of the mammary chain, although the others may also be affected. Local lymph node enlargement may become noticeable as well. A fluid discharge from the affected nipples may occur, and, if metastasis takes place, breathing difficulties, coughing, swollen limbs, vomiting, and/or diarrhea may arise.

The treatment of choice for any type of mammary tumor is surgical removal. This may involve simply removing the mass if only one location along the mammary chain is affected, or in the case of multiple locations, the entire gland or a large portion thereof may need to be removed. Regional lymph nodes are removed as well if metastasis is suspected. Upon biopsy of the affected tissue, subsequent chemotherapy is recommended if the tumor is deemed malignant.

Besides mammary adenocarcinomas, other adenomas/adenocarcinomas seen in older cats include *ceruminous gland tumors*, which affect the ears and ear canals, *pancreatic adenomas/adenocarcinomas, intestinal adenocarcinomas,* and *pituitary gland* and *adrenal gland adenomas* (causes of Cushing's disease in cats). In addition, adenomas affecting the thyroid glands (*thyroid adenomas*) in older cats are responsible for the development of hyperthyroidism (see page 104). Diagnosis of these various types of tumors is achieved through a combination of clinical signs, physical exam findings, radiography, ultrasonography, and surgical biopsy. Treatment for adenocarcinomas employs surgical removal, chemotherapy, and/or radiation therapy.

Squamous cell carcinomas (SCC) arise from the superficial epithelial cells comprising the skin. Areas of skin lacking pigment (such as that seen in cats with all-white hair coats or white spotting) and subject to repeated trauma, irritation, or ultraviolet radiation from the sun are especially susceptible to SCC development. The nose, sinuses, oral cavity, tonsils, lips, gums, tongue, teeth, eyelids, and external ear are the most common sites of occurrence in cats.

A squamous cell carcinoma may appear as a slightly raised mass, often with an ulcerated surface, or it may actually resemble a small bump or wart. As a rule, these tumors are slow to spread to other organs, yet usually readily invade surrounding tissue. Diagnosis is achieved through biopsy evaluation of the actual tumor. Surgery, cryotherapy, hyperthermia, and radiation therapy are the most effective ways to treat SCC in older cats.

Osteosarcoma (OSA) is the name given to a highly malignant tumor involving bone. This tumor is quite destructive in nature and metastasizes readily to other organs of the body, especially the lungs. Locally, bone destruction with infiltration of surrounding tissues occurs in most cases. The most common sites of involvement in the cat are the hind limbs and skull. Clinical signs associated with OSA include localized swelling, limb or facial deformity, and lameness. Coughing, breathing difficulties, and other signs related to internal organ involvement may also be seen if metastasis has occurred. Diagnosis can usually be made with clinical signs and with radiographs of the affected bones. Of course, biopsy evaluation is needed to confirm such a diagnosis.

Treatment for osteosarcomas involving the bones of the limbs involves aggressive surgical intervention, including amputation of the affected limb or special surgical techniques designed to preserve limb integrity while allowing for tumor removal. Chemotherapy should follow surgery to slow or eliminate metastatic disease.

Fibrosarcomas are malignant tumors arising from the fibrous tissue located just beneath the skin. They usually present as solitary, irregular masses on or protruding from the skin. Their surfaces may or

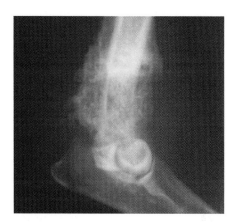

Osteosarcoma affecting the elbow region of a cat.

may not be ulcerated. Over 50 percent of all fibrosarcomas occur on the limbs. In addition, in rare instances, fibrosarcomas have been known to develop at sites of vaccine administration along the back and flank regions. When they occur, fibrosarcomas aggressively invade local tissue, and secondary metastasis to the lungs and lymph nodes is not uncommon.

Diagnosis of fibrosarcomas is made through biopsy evaluation. Treatment usually involves a combination of surgery (most important), radiation therapy, and cryotherapy.

Meningioma is the most prevalent neoplasia affecting the nervous system of cats. Originating from the thin membranes that cover the surface of the brain, meningiomas are usually benign in character, yet their growth within the enclosed space of the skull places tremendous pressure upon the brain tissue. The resulting clinical signs usually include depression, circling, seizures, restlessness, and behavioral disorders.

Table 23:
Common Tumors Affecting Older Cats

Tumor Type	Tissue/Organ Affected	Primary Mode(s) of Treatment*	Comments
Adenoma/ adenocarcinoma	Mammary glands; intestines; ear canals; pancreas; pituitary gland; adrenal gland; skin; ovaries; uterus; thyroid	S, C, R, Cr	Malignant tumors associated with glandular organs
Basal cell tumor	Skin	S, R	Most common skin tumor in cats
Chondrosarcoma	Bone; nasal cavity	S, R, C	Malignant tumor of cartilage
Fibrosarcoma	Connective tissue beneath the skin; oral cavity; nerves	S, R, Cr	May be induced by vaccines in some cats
Hemangiosarcoma	Skin	S, C, Cr	Rare in cats
Leukemia/ myelo- proliferative disorders	Blood; lymph nodes Bone marrow	C, I	Commonly associated with FeLV
Lipoma	Fatty tissue	S	Usually infiltrates into adjacent tissue
Lymphoma/ lymphosarcoma	Blood; lymph nodes; intestines; spleen; liver; kidneys; skin; eyes; brain; spinal cord; pancreas	C, I	Most common tumor seen in cats; frequently induced by FeLV
Mast cell sarcoma	Skin	S, R, C, Cr	Fourth most common skin tumor of cats; sometimes characterized by intense itching and allergic reaction
Melanoma	Skin; oral cavity	S, R	Often highly malignant and metastasizing; often highly pigmented
Meningioma	Brain	S	Most common tumor affecting the nervous system of cats
Metastatic bone tumor	Bone	S, C, R	Most often arises from mammary tumors

Table 23 (continued):
Common Tumors Affecting Older Cats

Tumor Type	Tissue/Organ Affected	Primary Mode(s) of Treatment*	Comments
Metastatic liver tumor	Liver	S, C, R	Most often arises from intestinal adenocarcinomas; lymphosarcoma
Metastatic lung tumor	Lungs	S, C, R	Usually arises from sarcomas; some carcinomas (mammary)
Multiple myeloma	Bone; bone marrow; blood	C	Caused by plasma cells, which are types of white blood cells; tumors often cause spontaneous fractures in affected bones
Osteosarcoma	Bone	S, C	Amputation is often treatment of choice
Papilloma; sebaceous adenoma	Skin; oral cavity; nasal cavity, eyelids; ears	S, Cr	Appear as wartlike growths on the skin and mucous membranes
Rhabdomyomas	Muscle tissue	S	Extremely rare in cats
Squamous cell carcinoma	Skin; oral cavity; eyelids	S, H, Cr, R	Second most common skin tumor in cats; white-haired, blue-eyed cats most prone
Transitional cell carcinoma	Bladder	S, C, R	Extremely rare in cats; malignant cells may be detected in urine

* S—Surgery; C—Chemotherapy; R—Radiation; Cr—Cryotherapy; I—Immunotherapy; H—Hyperthermia

Diagnosis of a meningioma can be made using radiographs of the skull or CT scans. Surgical removal is the treatment of choice for this particular tumor.

There are a multitude of other tumor types that occur with lower frequency in older cats. (For a summary of these tumors and modes of treatments, see Table 23.)

Chapter Six
Clinical Signs and Complaints

As your pet advances in years, you must become especially astute to changes in behavior or in physical anatomy and function that may signal the onset of disease. Your ability to recognize and distinguish actual disease conditions from normal age-related changes and to react accordingly is a critical key in extending your cat's life. Timing is of the essence when it comes to effective treatment or management of disease. The sooner a clinical sign is reported to your veterinarian, the better the chances are of identifying and halting the progression of a disease.

Clinical signs (symptoms) are not disease entities in themselves, but rather the outward manifestations of disease. The onset of symptoms may occur acutely (suddenly) or slowly and progressively over a period of time. In some instances, the underlying disease condition causing the clinical sign may be in advanced development before the symptom even appears. For example, pronounced weight loss, excessive thirst and urination, vom-

iting, and other signs linked to chronic kidney failure may not become readily apparent until at least 75 percent of the kidney tissue has been rendered nonfunctional. As a result, any delays in seeking out professional help once symptoms appear could turn an otherwise manageable condition into a life-threatening crisis.

Although the clinical signs and complaints presented in this section are among the more common encountered by owners of older cats, they are not all encompassing. In addition, the possible etiologies (causes) of each are certainly not limited to those listed. As a result, proper veterinary diagnosis of the actual underlying cause of your pet's clinical signs is essential.

Abdominal Pain

A cat with abdominal pain exhibits a tense abdomen that is noticeably tender to the touch. This is usually caused by abnormal pressure within or stretching of an organ or organs, or by actual rup-

Causes of Abdominal Pain in Older Cats

Abdominal tumor
Constipation
Feline infectious peritonitis (FIP)
Feline urologic syndrome (FUS)
Granuloma or abscess
Infectious gastroenteritis
Intestinal foreign body and/or
   obstruction
Kidney disease
Liver disease
Organ rupture due to trauma or
   neoplasia
Pancreatitis
Poisoning
Ulcers

ture of the organ. Cats suffering from acute abdominal pain will often exhibit a hunched, arched-back posture, with a reluctance to walk. When handled by their owners, they may become aggressive due to pain. Depending upon the organ(s) involved, abdominal pain may also be accompanied by vomiting, diarrhea, icterus, seizures, abdominal swelling, and shock.

Diagnosing the cause of abdominal pain involves the evaluation of a complete history and physical examination, blood profiles, and radiography or ultrasonography of the abdomen.

Immediate treatment for abdominal discomfort includes the use of injectable pain relievers and smooth muscle relaxants. In severe cases, intravenous fluid therapy and other supportive measures may be required, pending a diagnosis.

Abdominal Swelling

Abdominal swelling may or may not be accompanied by abdominal pain. In most cases, noticeable swelling in the abdomen of older cats is caused by fluid accumulation within the abdomen, or by a bloated or full stomach. The onset of the clinical sign may provide clues as to its origin. For instance, a sudden onset of abdominal swelling may be seen following ingestion of a meal, internal hemorrhage, or urinary obstruction. On the other hand, a slow, progressive onset is characteristic of heart failure, neoplasia, and obesity.

Apart from physical examination, identification of the cause of abdominal swelling is assisted

Cats experiencing abdominal pain will often have a "hunched up" appearance.

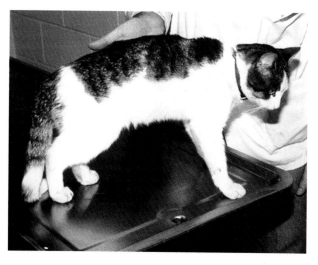

Severe fluid accumulation within the abdomen secondary to liver disease, leading to abdominal swelling.

through the use of radiographs, ultrasound, and/or laboratory blood analysis. In addition, a veterinarian may insert a needle into the abdominal cavity in order to remove and examine any fluid or material obtained under a microscope. Treatment approaches are based upon diagnostic conclusions.

Appetite, Increased (Polyphagia)

Polyphagia, a marked increase in appetite, has short-term health ramifications in cats that are not as significant as those seen with loss of appetite. However, its onset could be indicative of underlying disease and warrants due attention. In many instances, polyphagia can be induced when a cat is switched over to a ration designed for seniors. These diets are lower in calories than those designed for young and middle-aged adults, and if portion sizes are not adjusted with the changeover, caloric deprivation and subsequent polyphagia can result. A multitude of diseases can also cause polyphagia. As a result, a veterinary evaluation is required if this symptom is seen. Once a diagnosis is achieved, treatment can be directed at correcting the underlying cause.

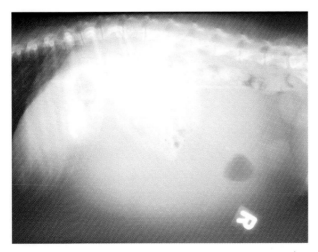

Appetite, Loss of

Anorexia is the medical term for loss of appetite. Although it is not unusual for a cat to go one or two days without eating, loss of appetite extending three days or beyond should be considered abnormal. Left untreated, this reduction in caloric intake can lead to a state of starvation. This, in turn, can lead to weight loss, wasting, diarrhea, anemia, poor wound healing, immunosuppression, and liver disease.

Diagnosing the underlying cause of anorexia involves the use of behavioral history, physical examination, laboratory blood analysis, and, if needed, radiography. A lasting cure, of course, is dependent upon the underlying cause and its treatability.

The ability to smell a ration plays an important role in appetite in cats, and any interruption or interference with the sense of smell will usually result in loss of appetite. This often occurs secondarily to viral upper respiratory infections and trauma to the nasal passages. In any case, restoring the sense of smell by controlling and removing nasal discharge and inflammation is a priority. Warming a ration to increase its aroma or feeding one of higher palatability can be used to stimulate the appetite of cats exhibiting loss of appetite. In especially tough cases, special medications, including B vitamins, anabolic steroids, and certain antianxiety medications

Causes of Anorexia (Loss of Appetite) in Older Cats

Abscess
Anemia
Cardiomyopathy
Dehydration
Dietary boredom
Fever
Gastrointestinal disease
Kidney disease
Liver disease
Loss of smell
Nausea
Neoplasia
Pain
Pancreatitis
Trauma
Upper respiratory infection

can be prescribed or employed by a veterinarian in an attempt to increase food consumption. If fever is causing or complicating the anorexia, anti-inflammatory medications given by injection work well in restoring appetite.

Breathing Difficulties

Breathing difficulties in older cats most commonly result from serious heart and/or lung disease, and pleural effusions. Noticeable respiratory distress may occur either upon the inhalation phase of breathing or the exhalation phase. Extreme care must be taken when handling respiratory-distressed

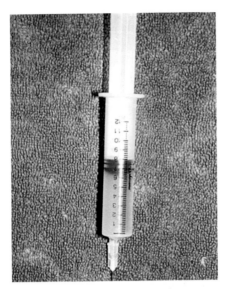

felines, because any degree of stress can lead to collapse.

Observation of breathing patterns, chest auscultation (utilizing a stethoscope), and chest radiographs

Causes of Breathing Difficulties in Older Cats

Allergic bronchitis (feline asthma)
Anemia
Heart disease and pulmonary edema
Heartworm disease (rare)
Neoplasia (FeLV associated)
Obesity
Pleural effusions (FIP)
Pneumonia
Pneumothorax
Respiratory foreign body
Rhinotracheitis
Trauma

are all useful in establishing a diagnosis. In addition, most cats suffering from breathing difficulties will be tested for FeLV and FIV, regardless of vaccination status. Often, nonspecific treatment must be initiated even before diagnostics can be performed. Such treatment can entail oxygen therapy, removal of any fluid accumulated within the chest using a needle and syringe or drainage tube, and medications designed to dilate airways and blood vessels and mobilize any fluid or edema out of the lungs. Once a diagnosis is achieved, specific treatment can then be added to the existing regimen.

Constipation

Constipation is a condition characterized by the inability to defecate with ease or regularity, resulting in fecal retention within the colon. *Tenesmus*, or straining to defecate, usually accompanies constipation due to the difficulty in passage. This dilemma tends to worsen over time, because the longer the feces is retained in the colon, the more moisture is reabsorbed by the colon, predisposing to even greater dryness and impaction. Other clinical signs seen with constipation include anxiousness, vocalizations while trying to eliminate, and a hunched-back appearance. In severe, long-standing cases of constipation, loss of appetite, vomiting, and dehydration can be seen. In cats, straining due to constipation must be differenti-

Causes of Constipation and Tenesmus in Older Cats

Anal sac impaction/infection
Drug therapy
Feline megacolon
Fluid imbalances/dehydration
Foreign matter in stool
Fractured pelvis
Hyperthyroidism
Intestinal parasites
Intestinal neoplasia
Intestinal obstruction
Spinal cord trauma

ated from urinary straining caused by FUS.

There are several potential causes of constipation in older cats. A conclusive diagnosis of the underlying cause can generally be made using a history of the problem, physical examination, stool evaluations, and radiographs of the abdomen. Initial treatment for constipation involves emptying the colon using soapy, warm water enemas. Sedation or anesthesia may be required for this procedure if the patient is in exceptional pain and/or excitable. Regardless of whether sedation is needed or not, only a veterinarian should administer enemas to cats. Never, under any circumstances, should an enema preparation designed for humans be used in a cat; such a preparation can cause rapid dehydration, electrolyte imbalances, and death.

For severe cases of constipation, intravenous fluid therapy may be required to restore water balance within the body and help normalize large intestinal function. Surgical intervention may be required in select cases to correct any underlying causes that may be present.

Long-term management procedures to prevent recurrences of constipation will depend upon the underlying cause of the disorder. Laxatives may be prescribed to help regulate the frequency of bowel movements. In addition, dietary adjustment, which can include increasing the amount of fiber in the ration, is an effective means of long-term management of constipation in older felines. Commercially available bran supplements or prescription cat foods containing higher amounts of fiber may be used to achieve this goal.

Coughing

Coughing is a reflex action initiated by stimulation of cough receptors located all along the respiratory tract. Because the possible causes of coughing in cats are so numerous, a stepwise approach to diagnostics is often required to narrow the field of possible causes. Historical information and patient characteristics are important in establishing a diagnosis. For instance, outdoor cats (especially those not kept current on vaccinations) have a greater propensity for developing coughs related to infectious diseases or parasites than do those

Causes of Coughing in Older Cats

Allergic bronchitis (feline asthma)
Cardiomyopathy (pulmonary edema)
Deep fungal infection
Infectious rhinotracheitis
Lungworms
Metastatic lung cancer
Pneumonia
Respiratory foreign body
Tonsillitis

kept indoors. Obesity can also predispose an older cat to coughing due to compression of fat on the respiratory system and due to stress placed on the immune system, predisposing to infectious diseases and tumors. Potential exposure to other ill cats is also important in the differential diagnosis of coughing. For example, introduction of a new kitten with upper respiratory disease into a household can pose a health threat to older cats, even those that are current on immunizations.

The character of a cough is also important in establishing a diagnosis. For instance, dry, hacking coughs can be seen with irritations involving the respiratory tract and lung tumors, whereas moist coughs characterized by a buildup of mucus or fluid may be seen with cardiomyopathy and pneumonia. Coughing that occurs mainly at night often has a failing heart as its source, as do coughs that occur after play or rigorous activity. Coughing that occurs after eating may signify a disease of the esophagus or mouth that is preventing normal passage of food into the stomach. Finally, a buildup of respiratory secretions secondary to allergies or feline asthma, or the presence of a foreign body in the oral cavity, esophagus, and/or trachea can cause a characteristic gagging cough and cyanosis (a condition of oxygen deprivation) in cats so affected.

Tests and procedures utilized in the search for a diagnosis of a cough include a thorough history, physical examination, CBC, biochemistry profiles, chest and neck radiographs, FeLV and FIV testing, ultrasonography, endoscopy, and/or microscopic examination of mucus and fluid expelled during a coughing episode.

Treatment of coughing in cats is dependent upon the underlying cause. Coughs with infectious origins are treated with antibiotics, nebulization therapy (inhalation of humidified and/or medicated air) and if nonproductive in nature, cough suppressants. When a cough is productive (one in which excessive respiratory secretions are expelled with each cough), cough suppressants should not be used, because an accelerated buildup of respiratory secretions and inflammatory debris within the lungs could result. Finally, for those coughs caused by heart disease, the use of appropriate therapy will help resolve the cough.

Diarrhea

Diarrhea is a clinical sign of intestinal disease that is characterized by an abnormal increase in the water content of the feces, resulting in an increased frequency of elimination and volume of feces. Diarrhea marked by an abrupt, explosive onset—acute diarrhea—may not be accompanied by weakness, fever, and/or loss of appetite. Depending upon treatment, it will usually run its course within three to five days. Most cases of acute diarrhea, such as those caused by dietary indiscretions, are self-limiting; that is, they will clear up on their own without specific treatment. However, for those cases persisting for more than 48 hours, or accompanied by other clinical signs, veterinary evaluation is required. A specific diagnosis and treatment are needed in these instances to prevent dehydration, malnutrition, and, in severe cases, shock.

Diarrhea that persists for more than 21 days, or recurs on a periodic basis, is called chronic diarrhea. These chronic or recurring bouts can cause malnourishment and stress in older cats, both of which can suppress the cat's immune system. Again, proper diagnosis of the underlying cause and treatment is required.

The potential causes of diarrhea in older cats are diverse and abundant. A good history of the problem will help the veterinarian pinpoint the location of the disorder. For instance, if a cat is exhibiting elimination urgency more than likely the diarrhea is originating in the large, rather than in the small, intestine. In addition, a black, tarry stool is usually indicative of small intestinal bleeding and inflammation, whereas red blood in the stool occurs with large intestinal inflammation. Potential exposure to other sick animals, foreign objects, or toxins is also important information that can help lead to a diagnosis.

The physical examination is another important tool for uncovering the source of diarrhea. For example, a dull, unthrifty hair coat could indicate a nutrient absorption or utilization disorder or internal parasites within the intestines. Furthermore, pronounced weight loss noted on exam usually indicates an

Causes of Diarrhea in Older Cats

Autoimmune disease
Bacterial intestinal infections
Deep fungal infections
Dietary indiscretions/changes
Food allergy
Intestinal parasites
Intestinal neoplasia
Intestinal obstruction
Intestinal foreign body
Kidney disease
Liver disease
Pancreatitis
Toxins/drugs
Viral intestinal infections

infection, neoplasia, or immune disorder affecting the small intestine, with varying degrees of dehydration and malnourishment. Finally, physical examination and abdominal palpation may detect obvious foreign bodies or masses involving the intestinal regions in diarrheic felines.

In addition to a physical exam, complete blood counts, serum biochemical profiles, FeLV and FIV testing, urinalysis, fecal exams, radiography, ultrasonography, and endoscopy may be needed to achieve an exact diagnosis. Treatment of acute diarrhea with no other accompanying clinical signs consists of restricting food intake for a minimum of 24 hours. After this period, feedings may be resumed using a bland, low-fat diet for five to seven days. Bismuth subsalicylate and other over-the-counter antidiarrheal mixtures should only be used under the directions and guidance of a veterinarian, because salicylates and other similar substances can be highly toxic to cats.

For acute cases of diarrhea that don't respond within 48 hours to the above treatments, or for those characterized by the presence of weakness, fever, loss of appetite, or other clinical signs, veterinary intervention is required. Intravenous fluid therapy may be needed if the diarrhea has resulted in clinical dehydration. In addition to specific treatments aimed at the diagnosed cause, antidiarrheal medications designed to regulate fluid levels and motility within the intestines, anti-inflammatory medications, and intestinal surface protectants such as kaolin may be prescribed.

Discharge: Nose, Eyes, Reproductive Tract, Ears, Skin

In veterinary medicine, *discharge* is the drainage of fluid or semifluid material from an external opening or wound. Discharges are responses to inflammation and/or buildup of fluid pressure within a tissue or organ space. The categories of discharges that can be seen in older cats include nasal discharges, ocular (eye) discharges, reproductive discharges, ear discharges, and dermatologic discharges.

The color and character of a discharge can narrow the possibilities when it comes to identifying the cause. Serous discharges are thin, clear, and sometimes sticky. These are often seen in response to allergies, viral infections, and irritation due to foreign matter. Mucoid discharges are mucuslike, often white to green in color, thick, and very stringy. These are sometimes seen in conjunction with or as a sequela to serous-type discharges, with the causes being very similar. Purulent discharges are characterized by the presence of pus. Very odorous, thick, and cream to green-brown in color, purulent discharges are seen

Causes of Discharges in Older Cats

Discharges involving the nose
Allergies (serous, mucoid)
Bacterial infection (purulent, sanguineous)
Fungal infection (purulent, sanguineous, hemorrhagic)
Tumor, polyp (purulent, sanguineous, hemorrhagic)
Trauma (hemorrhagic)
Foreign body (serous, mucoid, purulent, hemorrhagic)
Blood clotting disorder (hemorrhagic)
Periodontal disease (purulent, hemorrhagic)
Open socket due to tooth loss (purulent, hemorrhagic)
Viral infection (serous, sanguineous)

Discharges involving the eyes
Allergies (serous, mucoid)
Bacterial infection (purulent)
Foreign matter (serous, mucoid)
Neoplasia/cyst (mucoid, purulent, hemorrhagic)
Trauma (hemorrhagic, serous)
Viral infection (serous)

Discharges involving the reproductive tract
Bacterial infection (purulent, hemorrhagic)
Neoplasia/cyst (mucoid, purulent, hemorrhagic)
Tumor, polyp (purulent, sanguineous, hemorrhagic)
Vaginitis/metritis (purulent, hemorrhagic)

Discharges involving the ears
Bacterial infection (purulent, hemorrhagic)
Ear mites (black, crusty)
Trauma (hemorrhagic)
Yeast infection (brown, odorous)

Discharge involving the skin
Bacterial infection/abscess (purulent)
Fungal infection (brown, purulent, hemorrhagic, granular)

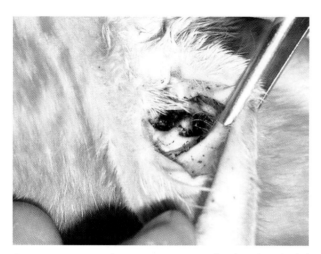

Ear discharge caused by mite infestation.

whenever pus-producing bacterial infections are present. These may be primary infections, or may occur secondarily to other insults. In addition, fast-growing tumors causing extensive tissue damage can predispose to purulent-type discharges. Finally, sanguineous and hemorrhagic discharges have blood as a component (the latter consisting almost entirely of blood) and are usually seen as a result of trauma, tumors, clotting disorders, poisonings, and certain infectious diseases. Such discharges can exist independently or in combination with other types. For example, a discharge that contains both mucus and pus is called a *mucopurulent discharge.* Similarly, a serous discharge that is blood tinged is referred to as a *serosanguineous discharge.*

Diagnosis of the underlying cause of a discharge will involve analysis of historical complaints of the problem, a complete physical examination, and appropriate laboratory tests. Oftentimes, microscopic examination of the discharge will lead a veterinarian to a diagnosis with no further laboratory workup required. However, in difficult cases, radiographs or endoscopic examinations may be necessary to pinpoint the exact cause.

Treatment for a discharge will be geared toward correcting the underlying cause. For instance, serous nasal discharges caused by allergies will often respond to nasal decongestants and anti-inflammatory medications. Purulent discharges signify the need for appropriate antibiotic therapy to bring the infection under control. Hemorrhagic discharges from the vagina of an intact female cat over eight years of age usually warrant an ovariohysterectomy. Discharges from the ears are usually caused by infectious agents or parasites, and need to be treated accordingly with topical antimicrobial or antiparasitic agents respectively.

Ear, Deafness In

See The Ears, page 140.

Eye, Blindness In

See The Eyes, page 134.

Eye, Redness or Cloudiness of

Inflammation involving the conjunctival membrane lining the eye

cause. If foreign body irritation is suspected, flushing the eye thoroughly with warm water will be of some benefit. If the corneal surface of the eye is not ulcerated, anti-inflammatory ointments and drops can be used to reduce inflammation and redness, whereas antibiotics are indicated in cases of infection and corneal ulcers. More aggressive therapy will be required for serious conditions such as uveitis and glaucoma to prevent permanent damage to the eye(s).

socket and the sclera (the white portion of the eyeball) creates the appearance of a "red eye" in cats. Inflammation usually is accompanied by squinting (photophobia) and a discharge, either serous or mucoid. Clear discharges are usually indicative of allergies and surface irritations; thicker mucoid discharges are seen with actual infections and foreign bodies. Apart from cataracts, a cloudy appearance to the eye may result from edema, scarring, and/or pigmentation of the cornea secondary to inflammation, corneal ulceration, or increases in eye pressures.

Careful ophthalmologic examinations, followed by special tests to check the integrity of the cornea and the pressure within the affected eye(s) will usually lead to a diagnosis. FeLV and FIV testing is certainly warranted, because both diseases can affect the eyes.

As always, treatment will be geared toward the underlying

Facial Swelling

Facial swelling can have a number of causes in older cats. The nature and location of the swelling is important for diagnostic purposes. For instance, semifirm to fluctuant localized swellings that are painful to the touch are likely to be abscesses or sites of bite or sting wounds. On the contrary, localized swellings that are firm or hard to the touch are usually caused by tumors, chronic infections, or enlarged lymph nodes. Lastly, diffuse, symmetrical swellings can most often be attributed to allergic reactions. Regardless of the cause, swellings involving the facial regions should be attended to promptly. Though most are associated only with pain and discomfort, some facial swellings can become life threatening if their development interferes with the normal flow of air through the nose and/or trachea.

The first step in obtaining a conclusive diagnosis of facial swelling is to rule out potential exposure to snakes, insects, or aggressive animals. A thorough physical exam is warranted, along with cytology of the swelling. Radiographs are useful in select instances as well. Treatment is selected based upon diagnostic findings. In allergic reactions, a combination of antihistamine and anti-inflammatory injections will alleviate an acute swelling quite effectively.

Fever

The normal temperature range for a cat should range anywhere from 100 to 103.2°F (37.8–39.5°C). Any elevation of temperature above the higher figure in the absence of previous exercise or rigorous activity should be considered abnormal. Cats exhibiting elevated temperatures will usually show signs of weakness, loss of appetite, and malaise. Other indications of fever

Causes of True Fever in Older Cats

Autoimmune disease
Drug therapy (tetracycline antibiotics)
Infections (bacterial, viral, fungal)
Inflammation due to disease or injury
Neoplasia

in cats may include shivering, piloerection (hair standing on end), curling up, and an active search for warm areas of the house.

It is important to differentiate a true fever from hyperthermia. Both conditions are characterized by elevated body temperatures but the causes of the two are very different. True fever occurs when the body readjusts its "thermostat" within the brain in response to inflammation, infection, or the release of certain chemicals. In cases of true fever, body temperature rarely exceeds 107°F (41.7°C). In contrast, hyperthermia results from the body being subjected to excessive muscular exertion or external heat sources.

Causes of Hyperthermia in Older Cats

Excitement/fear
Heat stroke
Overexertion
Seizures

For instance, increased muscle activity associated with seizures in older cats can quickly lead to a hyperthermic state. Heat stroke is a severe form of hyperthermia seen in cats exposed to high environmental temperatures. In some cases of heat stroke, body temperatures can elevate beyond 110°F (43.3°C). Obviously such a condition will lead to death if not recognized and treated promptly.

To obtain your cat's temperature, insert a plastic digital thermometer into its rectum for one to two minutes. Glass thermometers should not be used due to the danger of breakage. Although any elevation in temperature is significant, temperatures exceeding 105°F (40.6°C) should be considered medical emergencies and warrant immediate attention.

Treatment of true fever is geared towards treating the underlying cause once diagnosed. Anti-inflammatory medications designed to reduce the fever maybe administered by a veterinarian while the diagnostic workup is being performed. Aspirin can be extremely toxic to cats even in small dosages and should be administered only under the guidance and direction of a veterinarian. Under no circumstances should acetaminophen or ibuprofen be administered to cats. Both are highly toxic to felines and can kill quickly.

If hyperthermia is diagnosed or even suspected, whole body cooling is the only effective method of reducing body temperature. Immersing affected cats in ice water baths or administering alcohol baths will help rapidly lower body temperatures to safe levels. Cold water enemas may even be given to expedite the process. These procedures should be continued until a body temperature of 103°F (39.4°C) is achieved. Once this is accomplished, cooling procedures should be discontinued to prevent accidental hypothermia.

Incoordination, Falling, and Circling

Incoordination, falling, and circling activities are all usually caused by disorders affecting the nervous system in some way. All may exhibit either sudden or progressive onsets, and may appear in conjunction with one another. Falling and incoordination must be differentiated from true weakness, which can have an entirely different set of causes (see Weakness, page 179). The former result from a deficiency in proprioception, which is the nervous system's ability to coordinate limb, eye, and body movements with sensory input. Circling is usually caused by inflammation or direct pressure placed upon the brain.

Care must be taken when interacting with cats exhibiting any of these clinical signs, because disorientation could lead to sudden aggressiveness. Diagnostic efforts

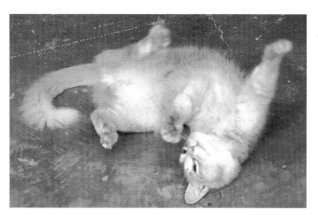

Falling and circling behavior secondary to a nervous system infection.

should be directed at the brain, spinal cord, and/or ears. Nonspecific treatments for incoordination, falling, and circling include strict confinement to prevent self-injury, sedatives, and anti-inflammatory medications, pending a conclusive diagnosis.

Causes of Incoordination, Falling, and/or Circling in Older Cats

Ear infection
FeLV/ FIV
FIE
FIP
Fracture
Infection involving nervous system
Inflammation of brain or spinal cord
Poisoning
Seizure
Toxoplasmosis
Trauma involving nervous system
Vestibular disease

Causes of Jaundice in Older Cats

Bile duct obstruction
Gall bladder disease
Internal bleeding and/or destruction of red blood cells
Liver disease

Jaundice (Icterus)

Jaundice, or icterus, is a clinical sign characterized by a yellow-orange discoloration of, among other things, the skin, mucous membranes, tissues, and organs. It is the result of elevated levels of bile pigments in the bloodstream. When present, it represents serious clinical disease and warrants prompt diagnosis and treatment of the underlying cause.

Lameness

Lameness is defined as the inability or reluctance to bear complete weight on one or more limbs. There are various degrees of lameness that can be observed, the severity of which can help lead to a diagnosis. For instance, a lameness in which the pet refuses to bear weight on the affected limb is usually indicative of a bone fracture or a joint dislocation. Older cats affected with a non-weight-bearing lameness will usually carry the affected limb close to the body with all joints flexed. A lameness that involves only a partial loss in function, sometimes referred to as a limp, can be caused by cat bite abscesses, minor fractures, and a multitude of other conditions.

A thorough history of the lameness will expedite the diagnostic process. It should include when the lameness was first noticed, the time of day the lameness is most noticeable, if it had a sudden or progressive onset, if the pet has experienced any trauma or interaction with aggressive cats within the past four to six weeks, and if there have been other changes in activity or behavior occurring along with the lameness. In addition a thorough veterinary orthopedic examination should be performed. During this examination, a veterinarian should be able to ascertain the exact location of the lameness, its extensiveness, and possibly its cause. For example, swelling, bruising, and pain noted at any point along a bone or joint often indicates that a fracture or ligament tear is present. Hard masses beneath the skin overlying and/or involving a bone or joint may lead a clinician to suspect a tumor or chronic infection.

Such histories and physical examination findings can lead to a tentative diagnosis of the cause of a lameness. However, radiographs, joint fluid analysis, biopsy procedures, and other laboratory tests may be needed to turn a tentative diagnosis into a definitive one.

Treatment for lameness will depend upon a conclusive diagno-

Causes of Lameness in Older Cats

Arthritis
Bruised or traumatized footpad
Cat fight abscess
Deep fungal infection
Degenerative joint disease
Foreign body penetration
Fracture
Hip dislocation
Hyperparathyroidism
Infections involving
  bones/joints/muscles
Joint sprain or strain
Ligament tear
Muscle trauma/bruising
Neoplasia

---

sis. For minor ligament sprains and muscle strains, as well as arthritic flare-ups, three to five days of forced rest combined with the administration of an anti-inflammatory pain reliever by a veterinarian will help to resolve minor lameness. Other causes will need to be addressed with medications and corrective procedures specific for the condition in question.

Odors: Body, Breath

Bad odors associated with older cats usually result from disease conditions that require veterinary attention. Careful examination of the oral cavity, skin, and hair coat will often reveal the source of the problem. In some cases, more in-depth

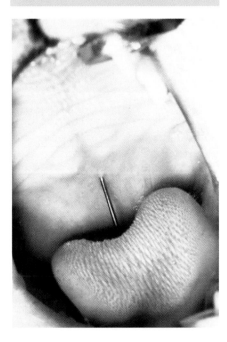

Foreign bodies in the mouth such as this needle can cause foul breath.

diagnostics may be required. If the underlying condition is properly diagnosed and treated, the unpleasant odor can usually be lessened or eliminated.

Paralysis

Paralysis affecting older cats can be divided into two types: sensory paralysis and motor paralysis. *Sensory paralysis* is characterized by loss of touch and pain sensation in the affected portions of the body. This type of paralysis is serious, because it can predispose to self-mutilation. In felines, sensory paralysis is usually accompanied by flaccid *motor paralysis*. With flaccid motor paralysis, the muscles responsible for movement fail to receive nervous impulses and are therefore rendered nonfunctional. In contrast, spastic motor paralysis is characterized by muscular rigidity and spasticity caused by uncontrolled and continuous nervous impulses to the muscles. With such a paralysis, the limbs and neck assume extended rigid positioning, making locomotion impossible. Spastic motor paralysis is most commonly seen with malicious poisonings. It also plays a role in the painful manifestation of thromboembolism seen in felines suffering from cardiomyopathy.

Paralysis may also affect certain internal organs if the nerves innervating these organs are disrupted or damaged. For instance, paralysis of the bladder or colon will result in the over-accumulation of wastes with these organs. In addition, paralysis can also play a role in the development of megacolon in cats.

Diagnosing the specific cause of paralysis requires a good history (including potential exposure to poisons), physical examination, and other diagnostic tests deemed necessary, including those specific for nervous system maladies. Treatment will be determined by the underlying cause. Drugs to reduce inflammation are indicated if trauma or other inflammatory disorders are responsible for the paralysis. In addition, muscle relaxants may be indicated in cases of spastic paralysis. Finally, in instances where sensory paralysis has affected a limb, amputation may be required to prevent self-mutilation and subsequent gangrene formation.

Regurgitation

See Vomiting, page 177.

Salivation, Excessive

Excessive salivation, or drooling, is often seen in older cats in response to the consumption of (or even anticipation of) an undesirable or irritating substance or object, such as medications, insects, and flea sprays. It is also a clinical sign of disease affecting either the oral cavity, esophagus, or stomach, and can occur secondary to seizures and other illnesses of the nervous system. Diagnosis of an underlying cause begins with careful examination of the oral cavity for any obvious abnormalities, and then, if needed, proceeding with specific testing procedures aimed at identifying other potential causes. As always, treatment will be customized according to the diagnosis. In the case of excessive salivation caused by the consumption of medications, plants,

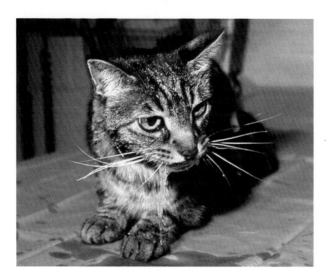

Excessive salivation resulting from the administration of oral medication.

insects, or other irritants, rinsing the mouth with copious amounts of water will serve to dilute the noxious substance and diminish this clinical sign. If a foreign object is lodged between the teeth or in the gums, tweezers can be used to manually extract the object, if the cat allows.

Seizures

A *seizure* is defined as uncontrollable behavior or muscle activity caused by an abnormal increase in nervous system activity. Seizures in older cats can occur with varying degrees; although a full-blown convulsion is usually envisioned, seizures should be suspected anytime a cat exhibits unusual or unexplained behavioral changes.

Depending upon the underlying cause, seizures can be continuous and unrelenting, as seen in certain types of poisonings, or sporadic and of short duration, as in cases of true epilepsy. The duration of the actual seizure episode is directly proportional to its danger. Typically, seizure episodes lasting over three minutes should be regarded as medical emergencies, warranting prompt veterinary attention.

In older cats, seizure activity must be differentiated from *syncope*, which refers to a loss of consciousness caused by oxygen deprivation to the brain. The two most common causes of syncope in mature felines include cardiomyopathy and anemia. These cats may appear fine one moment, then suddenly collapse and lose consciousness as a result of oxygen deficiency. Such an episode is often mistaken for a seizure.

The typical epileptic seizure has three distinct phases. The preictal phase is characterized by anxiety and restlessness. Next, the ictal phase or true seizure, is evidenced by recumbency, uncontrolled muscular contractions and eye movements, and spontaneous urination and/or defecation. The postictal phase following the true seizure is characterized by staggering, depression, confusion, and exhaustion, and usually lasts anywhere from 15 minutes to 6 hours.

As with other symptoms, diagnosis of the cause of a seizure is based upon analysis of the characteristics and frequency of the seizure activity, a physical examination, and appropriate laboratory tests, including a complete blood profile and urinalysis. If no underlying cause can be pinpointed for recurring seizures, a tentative diagnosis of idiopathic epilepsy is usually made. Although not common in felines, idiopathic epilepsy can show up at any age, and may last only a short while before permanently disappearing.

To prevent seizures from recurring, treatment must be geared toward correcting the underlying cause. When a cause cannot be discovered, or when the underlying disease is incurable, anticonvulsant medication such as diazepam or phenobarbital may be necessary to control seizure activity. Initially, frequent adjustments to the dosages of these medications may be necessary in an attempt to discover the ideal dose that can control seizures, yet cause minimal depression in the patient. In addition, because anticonvulsant medica-

tions can place undo stress on the liver, older cats receiving such drugs should have a liver function test performed at least once a year.

If your pet suffers from a seizure, do not attempt to intervene or hold the cat down during the ictal phase. To do so could cause injury to your cat and to you as well! Instead, throw a thick blanket or towel over the cat and "wait out" the seizure. Once completed, confine the cat to a small bathroom or a travel kennel until the disorientation associated with the postictal phase has disappeared. If the ictal phase of the seizure has extended beyond three minutes, wrap your pet securely in the blanket, using extreme caution not to be bitten, and transport it in this way to your veterinarian.

Skin, Dry and Flaky

See Seborrhea page 126.

Skin: Hair Loss (Alopecia) and Itching

Hair loss due to the presence of disease may be differentiated from hair loss caused by normal shedding by the appearance of bald patches of skin. In older cats, alopecia may occur secondary to inflammation or changes within hair follicles caused by underlying disease, or to relentless chewing and scratching by the cat itself.

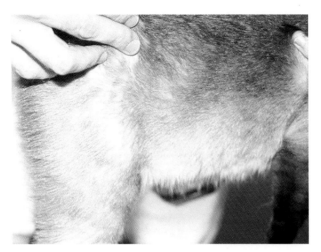

Alopecia in an older cat caused by allergies.

The distribution of the hair loss can provide valuable clues as to the underlying cause. For example, alopecia that is symmetrical in appearance (affecting both sides of the body equally) is usually caused by disturbances originating within the body, including allergies, nutritional deficiencies, and endocrine diseases. In contrast, patchy, random hair loss is usually seen with infections or parasites. The presence or absence of itching along with the alopecia is also significant when determining a diagnosis. Itching results from inflammation within the skin and/or hair follicles, and is usually seen along with hair loss. However, hair loss can also be seen in the absence of itching. In such instances, the underlying cause is either a hormonal imbalance, nutritional disorder, stress, ringworm, and neurodermatitis.

Once a diagnosis has been established, treatment of the underlying disorder will reverse most cases of alopecia. However, hair regrowth may be slow or may not occur at all if scarring has taken place within the skin and hair follicles, or if the underlying disease condition cannot be medically managed.

Anti-inflammatory medications, special diets, medicated shampoos, and topical moisturizing sprays may all be prescribed to discourage itching in cats while encouraging hair regrowth. Daily brushing will also stimulate hair growth and replacement while helping to soothe itchy skin.

Skin: Lumps and Masses on or Beneath

The appearance of a mass or lump on or beneath the skin in an older cat warrants prompt veterinary attention. Certainly the first thought that comes to mind is cancer, yet this is not always the case. There are several conditions that may appear as a neoplasia, yet are entirely different in origin. *Granulomas* represent a type of immune response mounted by the cat's body in response to a foreign body, fungi, or certain types of bacteria. Consisting of an accumulation of inflammatory cells, granulomas are well defined, symmetrical, and self-limiting as far as growth is concerned. *Cysts* are fluid or debris-filled sacs that may arise spontaneously or in conjunction with other diseases. True abscesses are caused by localized regions of bacterial infection. Soft, fluctuant, and painful to touch, abscesses are usually accompanied by fever and some degree of malaise in affected cats. *Hematomas* and *seromas* are painful, fluctuant masses resulting from leakage of blood or serum, respectively, from damaged blood vessels. Trauma to the skin and subcutaneous tissue can result in hematoma or seroma formation beneath the skin of the affected region. Finally, fibrous nodular scarring can occur secondary to foreign body penetration or most commonly, following vaccine administrations. Usually no bigger than a marble, these nodules will, with time, usually regress on their own. However, this regression should be monitored, because in rare instances, these fibrous nodules can become cancerous.

Causes of Lumps or Masses on or Beneath the Skin in Older Cats

Abscess
Cyst
Fibrous nodular scar
Granuloma
Hematoma/seroma
Swollen lymph node(s)
Tumor, benign or malignant

Identification of a mass or lump can be achieved through the use of cytology. If neoplasia is suspected, an actual biopsy will be required as well. The primary treatment for the majority of lumps or masses on or beneath the skin is surgical removal or drainage. In the case of abscesses, surgical drainage along with appropriate antibiotic therapy will be required for a cure.

Sneezing

Sneezing is a reflex act that is initiated by irritation within a portion of the respiratory system, namely the nasal cavity and surrounding tissues. A nasal discharge may or may not accompany sneezing episodes. In identifying the underlying cause of sneezing, a number of procedures are used. Apart from a standard physical examination and blood analysis, direct visual examination of the nasal passages while a cat is under sedation is the most valuable tool in this diagnostic

Allergic rhinitis
Feline infectious rhinotracheitis
Fungal infection
Nasal polyp or tumor
Nasal foreign body

process. At that time, samples of nasal secretions may be obtained for microscopic review, and radiographs of the nasal passages taken if necessary.

Sneezing caused by an infection within the nasal passages may be managed through the use of appropriate antimicrobial medications. Tumors and polyps involving the nasal passages are often treated with surgery and/or radiation to

**Causes of Increased
Thirst/Excessive Urination
in Older Cats**

Cushing's disease
Diabetes mellitus
Drug therapy (corticosteroids)
Feline urologic syndrome
Glomerulonephritis
Hyperthyroidism
Increase in physical activity
Kidney disease
Liver disease
Mineral/electrolyte imbalances
Poisoning
Stress
Uterine infection (pyometra)

help achieve remission and alleviate sneezing. In cases of sneezing caused by allergies, antihistamines and anti-inflammatory medications are usually effective at controlling clinical signs.

Thirst, Excessive

See Urination, Excessive, below.

Urination, Excessive

Polyuria/polydipsia (PU/PD) is defined as an abnormal elevation in urine output (PU) and an abnormal increase in water consumption (PD). PU/PD is a fairly common complaint seen by veterinarians with regard to older pets. Special laboratory tests using urine samples and blood serum can determine the filtration rate of the kidneys and their ability to conserve water within the body. Once polyuria/polydipsia is determined to exist, the underlying cause must itself be uncovered before effective treatment can be performed.

Urination: Incontinence

Urinary incontinence is a clinical sign associated with diseases affecting the urinary system and the nervous system. It is characterized by the inability of an older cat to control the flow of urine from the bladder. Incontinence may appear as a sudden, unexpected flow of urine, or as a continuous urine drip. Cats that are incontinent usually experience irritation and inflammation affecting the external genitalia and surrounding skin due to urine scalding and excessive licking.

Because the potential causes of the incontinence are so numerous, diagnosis of the underlying source can be difficult. Tests that focus both on the urinary and nervous systems will be needed to root out the cause. As with other symptoms, treatment of urinary incontinence will depend upon this cause. Antibiotics, anti-inflammatories, and medications designed to increase sphincter tone within the lower portion of the urinary tract have all been used to treat the incontinent cat.

Urination: Straining (Stranguria)

Apparent difficulty in voiding urine is a clinical sign of lower urinary tract disease. Over-distension of the bladder wall due to urine filling will stimulate an abnormal urge to urinate, as will irritation and inflammation affecting the bladder and urethral linings. Bloody urine may also be noted in cats straining to urinate, either due to the underlying disease or secondary to the excessive straining itself. Often, crystals that have formed within the urine as a result of FUS will nick and cut the inner surfaces of the bladder and urethra, creating an intense urge to urinate, even though actual urine may not be voided.

For those cats exhibiting stranguria, a determination must be made as to whether or not the bladder is full or empty. Stranguria accompanied by an empty bladder often signifies inflammation in the absence of an obstruction. In these instances, treatment of the underlying cause and use of smooth muscle relaxants can provide relief to a distressed pet. However, cats exhibiting stranguria, yet having a full bladder, could be suffering from an obstruction. If an obstruction is indeed causing the bladder to overfill, the stranguria will be accompanied by a painful abdomen and intense restlessness. Prompt urinary catheterization is needed to restore urine flow in these instances. If this is neglected, kidney failure, bladder rupture, and/or death could result.

Vomiting

Vomiting is the forceful expulsion of stomach contents out through

Causes of Vomiting in Older Cats

Abdominal neoplasia
Bacterial gastrointestinal infections
Brain disorders
Diabetes mellitus
Dietary indiscretions/changes
Feline panleukopenia
Feline urologic syndrome
FeLV/FIV
Food allergies
Gastrointestinal obstruction
Hairballs
Ingestion of a foreign body
Intestinal parasites
Kidney disease
Liver disease
Pyometra
Stomach ulcers
Stress
Toxins/drugs
Vestibular disorders

the mouth. This act must be differentiated from *regurgitation*, which is the passive expulsion of food from the esophagus. Regurgitation is caused by disorders involving the esophagus, not the stomach.

Vomiting is a reflex act resulting from stimulation of receptors in the brain and various organs throughout the body. Stimulation of these receptors can result from inflammation, irritation, distension, pressure, or toxins. Multiple vomiting episodes usually indicate serious underlying disease, and can quickly lead to electrolyte imbalances, dehydration, and shock. As a result, an underlying cause must be positively identified as rapidly as possible so that proper treatment can be instituted. Vaccination history, parasite prevention, and potential exposure to sick animals, toxins, drugs, and/or foreign bodies are all important information that can help lead to a diagnosis. In most cases, a thorough physical examination and laboratory workup are needed to uncover the exact cause of the vomiting and any secondary complications, such as dehydration, that may be present. Examples of appropriate laboratory work include complete blood counts, serum biochemical evaluations, fecal examination for internal parasites, radiographs (including contrast studies using barium swallows) and endoscopy. Exploratory surgery may also be required if these measures fail to pinpoint a diagnosis.

Specific treatment of a vomiting cat is dependent upon the underlying cause. For uncomplicated cases in which vomiting occurs no more than twice, withholding food and water for at least 24 hours often allows the body to recover on its own. However, if multiple episodes occur, vigorous treatment is required. This includes intravenous fluid therapy to correct and/or prevent dehydration and electrolyte imbalances. Antivomiting medications, as well as antibiotics to control secondary infections, may be necessary as well.

Weakness

Weakness as a clinical sign can arise from disorders involving a number of body systems, including the circulatory, respiratory, nervous, musculoskeletal, and/or endocrine systems. Episodes of weakness are often shrugged off as a normal consequence of aging or arthritis when, in reality, a serious medical condition may be the source. Intensities of these bouts of weakness can range anywhere from moderate weakness to actual collapse. The duration of the weakness episodes can often provide valuable clues as to the underlying cause. For instance, episodes lasting less than one minute are often related to heart and lung disease. Incidents lasting over one minute but less

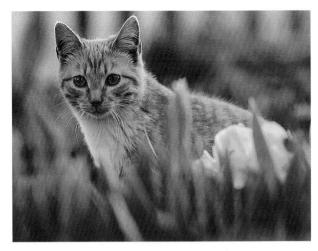

than five can often be attributed to seizure activity. Persistent, continuous weakness can result from neurological, endocrine, or musculoskeletal disorders, not to mention severe heart disease, anemia, and FeLV/FIV.

Because weakness is a nonspecific sign with a multitude of potential causes, a careful step-by-step approach to diagnostics is indicated. Starting with a thorough history and physical exam, diagnostic protocol may extend to laboratory testing of the blood, urine, and stool, ECGs, radiographs, ultrasound, FeLV/FIV testing, and a variety of other specialized tests. Once a cause is uncovered, appropriate treatment may be administered.

Causes of Weakness in Older Cats

Anemia
Arthritis
Dehydration
FeLV/FIV
Fever
Heart disease
Kidney disease
Low blood glucose
Malnourishment
Neoplasia
Pleural effusion
Poisoning
Spinal cord disease
Thromboembolism

Weight Loss and Wasting (Cachexia)

In cats, a progressive loss of body weight in the absence of a

Causes of Weight Loss and Wasting in Older Cats

Chronic infections
Diabetes mellitus
Exocrine pancreatic
 insufficiency
FeLV/FIV
FIP
Gastrointestinal parasites
Heart disease
Hyperthyroidism
Kidney disease
Liver disease
Maldigestion of food
Neoplasia
Persistent fever
Starvation
Stomatitis

predetermined weight loss program could signify the presence of an underlying disease. The term *cachexia* is used to describe weight loss and wasting occurring secondary to disease. The potential causes of progressive weight loss and wasting (cachexia) in older cats are numerous. A thorough medical history, physical examination, laboratory workup, and radiographs can all be utilized to pinpoint the cause of the problem.

Once a proper diagnosis has been made, specific treatment can be then undertaken to cure or manage the underlying disorder. In addition, high-energy diets, food supplements, anabolic steroids, and exercise may all be prescribed to help reverse a cat's cachexia.

Chapter Seven

Select First Aid Techniques for Older Cats

A s your cat grows older, the chances increase that you may be faced with an emergency situation brought about by injury or illness. If you suddenly find yourself in such a situation, don't panic! Remember that the purpose of any type of first aid is to stabilize your pet as much as possible until veterinary care can be obtained. Begin by assessing whether or not a life-threatening situation exists. Cessation of breathing, loss of pulse or heartbeat, extensive bleeding and trauma, poisoning, shock, and dehydration can all be classified as life-threatening circumstances and warrant the prompt rendering of first aid.

Always use caution when interacting with injured or ill cats, for they may exhibit aggressiveness if in pain or distress. If in doubt, consider draping a thick blanket or towel over your cat's head or donning heavy-duty gloves prior to handling or transporting it. Special muzzles designed for cats are also available from pet supply houses and should be purchased ahead of time in case such an emergency should arise.

Once first aid has been initiated, attention should be directed toward transporting your cat to your veterinarian as soon as possible. Be sure to call your veterinary office beforehand to describe your pet's condition and give your estimated time of arrival. This will enable them to make the necessary preparations needed to provide swift emergency care upon your arrival. Note: If you suspect that your cat may have suffered neck or spinal injury, transport it on a board or window screen to keep from aggravating the injury.

Artificial Respiration

Artificial respiration should be performed if your cat has stopped breathing. To determine whether or not this has occurred, observe the

Table 24: Normal Physiologic Values for Cats

- Temperature (degrees Fahrenheit)   100–103.2
- Pulse (beats per minute)   120–200
- Respirations (per minute)   20–30

chest for breathing movements or hold a mirror in front of your pet's nose. If your pet is breathing, condensation should be noted on the mirror surface. If your cat is not breathing:

- Determine if a heartbeat or pulse is present. If not, be prepared to integrate external heart massage with artificial respiration.
- Clear the mouth of any vomitus, blood, debris, or foreign objects, and pull the tongue straight out.
- Closing the mouth with the tongue still extended, place your mouth over your pet's nose and blow air into the nostrils until you see the chest expand.

Giving a pill to a cat.

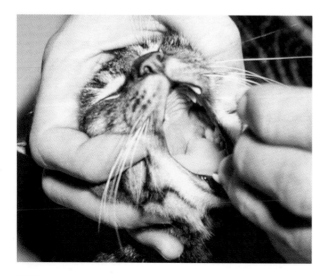

- Release the seal, allowing your cat to exhale.
- Repeat this sequence once every five seconds until your cat is breathing on its own or until veterinary care is obtained.

External Heart Massage

If a heartbeat or pulse cannot be seen, felt, or heard, then external heart massage must be initiated in conjunction with artificial respiration. To begin, first perform artificial respiration, and then:

- Position your cat on its right side.
- Grasp the lower portion of the chest with your hand, covering the front one third of the rib cage just behind the elbow. The palm of your hand should be adjacent to the sternum (breastbone).
- Using a quick, firm, and upward motion with your fingers, compress the chest 1 to 2 inches (2.5–5.1 cm), then release.
- Repeat the compressions at a rate of two per second. After every ten compressions, perform artificial respiration. Continue this process until veterinary assistance is obtained.

Bleeding

If your cat is bleeding profusely, immediately apply direct pressure to the source of the hemorrhage. Any readily available absorbable material or object, including gauze, towels, or shirts, can be used as a compress. Pressure should be applied at the source for no less than five minutes. If bleeding still persists secure the compress using gauze, a belt, pantyhose, or a necktie and seek veterinary help immediately. If an extremity is involved, applying pressure to the inside, upper portion of the affected leg will also reduce blood flow to the limb. If needed, a tourniquet—made with a belt, a necktie, or pantyhose—may be applied just above the wound. Use a pencil, ruler, or wooden spoon to twist and tighten the tourniquet until bleeding has been minimized. To prevent permanent damage to the limb, be sure you are able to pass one finger between the tourniquet and the skin without too much effort. In addition, release tourniquet pressure for 30 seconds every 10 to 15 minutes (applying direct pressure in its stead) until veterinary care is obtained.

Poisonings

General symptoms associated with poisoning in cats include vomiting, diarrhea, unconsciousness, seizures, abdominal pain, excessive salivation, panting, and/or shock.

Common sources of poisoning in older cats include houseplants, rodent poisons, insecticides, ethylene glycol (antifreeze), and drugs (aspirin, acetaminophen).

The goal of first aid treatment for poisoning is to dilute or neutralize the poison as much as possible prior to veterinary intervention.

If the poison originated from a container, always read and follow the label directions concerning accidental poisoning. In addition, be sure to take the label and container with you to your veterinarian. If a label is not available, then follow these guidelines:

- If your cat has ingested a caustic or petroleum-based substance, or if it is severely depressed, having a seizure, or unconscious, waste no time in seeking veterinary help. Treatment in these instances should be administered only under a veterinarian's guidance.

- For other ingested poisons, induce vomiting using 1 teaspoon of hydrogen peroxide (will cause intense salivation). Repeat the dosage of hydrogen peroxide in five minutes if needed.

- Following evacuation of the stomach, administer 1/2 cup of water orally to help dilute any remaining poison.

- If available, administer activated charcoal (mix 25 grams of powder in water to form a slurry, then administer 10 to 15 ml) or whole milk (1/2 cup) to help deactivate any residual poison.

Table 25:
At-Home Medications That Can Be Used for First Aid Purposes

If possible, always consult your veterinarian before giving anything orally to your older cat, especially if other medications are currently being given.

Administering oral tablets or capsules: Open your cat's mouth by placing one hand over the top of the muzzle, with your thumb and forefingers placed just behind the upper canine teeth. Slowly tilt your pet's head back, pressing inward and upward with your thumb and forefingers as you go. With your other hand placed at the very front of the lower jaw and holding the pill or capsule, separate the jaws and insert the pill as far back on the tongue as possible. Closing the mouth and lowering the head, gently stroke your pet's throat until you feel a swallow or until your cat licks its nose.

Administering oral liquids: Holding the cat's head as you would to administer a pill, insert the syringe, dropper, or spoon containing the medication into the mouth, slowly expelling the liquid once inside. Tilt your pet's head back to prevent the medication from escaping. Gently stroke the neck region until you feel a swallow.

Note: Following administration of a pill or liquid, some cats may salivate profusely in response to the medication. This is no cause for alarm and should subside within several minutes.

Medication	Indication	Dosage
3 percent hydrogen peroxide	To induce vomiting; general wound cleanser	1 teaspoon
Diphenhydramine	Mild cough; allergic reactions	0.5 mg per pound (use only on approval by your veterinarian)
Kaolin and pectin	Mild diarrhea	Use only under the direction of a veterinarian
Syrup of ipecac	To induce vomiting	1/4 teaspoon

Medication	Indication	Dosage
Milk of magnesia	Vomiting; constipation; deactivate poisons	1 teaspoon per 5 pounds body weight mixed with water
Activated charcoal	Poison deactivation	25 to 50 grams of powder mixed with water; give 1 ml per pound orally
Petroleum jelly	Constipation; hairballs	1/2 teaspoon per 10 pounds
Aloe vera	Burns; skin irritations	As needed

- If the poison was applied to the skin, flush the affected areas with copious amounts of water. If the offending substance is oil-based, a quick bath using water plus a mechanic's hand cleaner or a dishwashing liquid should be given to remove any remaining residue.
- In all instances of poisoning, specific antidotes may be available at your veterinarian's office. As a result, always seek out professional care following initial first aid efforts.

In addition to the above conditions, dehydration and circulatory shock are two more deadly situations that you may face in an emergency situation. However, because first aid measures for these two conditions are limited in scope, prompt veterinary intervention is going to be necessary to spare the life of your pet.

Circulatory shock is a life-threatening condition that can result from, among other things, severe trauma, pain, dehydration, or organ malfunction. With shock, specific physiological reactions impair blood circulation throughout the body, depriving organs and tissues of much needed oxygen and nutrients.

Signs of shock include recumbency; a rapid heart rate; a weak pulse; cold, pale mucous membranes; a dry, shriveled tongue;

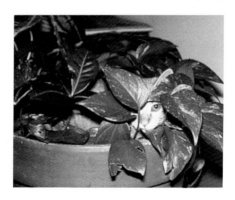

Houseplants can be a major source of poisoning in older cats.

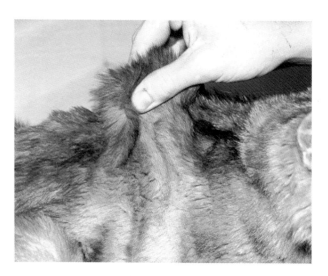

Checking for dehydration in a cat.

Dehydration in cats is characterized by weight loss, dry gums and mucous membranes, sunken eyeballs, protrusion of the third eyelids, and weakness. The skin of affected cats will lose its elasticity, which can be tested by gently lifting the skin along the back, then releasing it. If the skin fails to return to its normal position within one second, then a state of dehydration exists. As blood thickens and organs dehydrate due to the loss of fluids and electrolytes, circulatory shock and organ failure can ensue.

Some of the instigators of dehydration in older cats include food and water deprivation, burns, bleeding, vomiting, diarrhea, excessive panting, prolonged fever, kidney disease, endocrine disturbances, and certain types of drug therapy.

weakness; panting; a subnormal body temperature; and/or unconsciousness.

To reverse circulatory shock and preserve life, intravenous fluid and shock medication need to be instituted as fast as possible by a trained veterinarian. At-home first aid should include controlling any predisposing hemorrhage, conserving body temperature by wrapping your pet in a warm towel or blanket, reducing environmental stress, and transporting your cat to your veterinarian as quickly as possible.

If you suspect that your pet is dehydrated, seek veterinary care at once. Do not try to treat this condition at home. Only intravenous fluid replacement will effectively reverse the dehydration in a timely manner and lessen or prevent its deleterious effects upon internal organs.

Chapter Eight
Euthanasia and Your Older Cat

With pets today living longer than ever before, it is important for pet owners to confront the issue of euthanasia (what it is, how it is performed, and when it becomes necessary) before it suddenly and unexpectedly confronts them. Although it is an uncomfortable subject, preparing for its possibility will help lessen the stress and guilt you may experience if ever faced with such a decision concerning your devoted companion.

The term *euthanasia* refers to the purposeful and humane induction of unconsciousness and subsequent death. In veterinary medicine, this is usually accomplished through the use of special injectable formulations of anesthetic agents, such as sodium pentobarbital. Swift and painless, these agents induce death in a matter of seconds.

When does euthanasia become a consideration? Often, veterinarians are presented with cats for euthanasia that are perfectly healthy, except for personality (other than aggressiveness) or physical defects that make them "inconvenient" to their

owners. Others are brought in by relatives of a deceased person or of someone who has moved away. They claim that the pet would not be happy with anyone else and that therefore it should be put to sleep. These pets are not candidates for euthanasia and veterinarians should not be expected to honor such requests. Alternatives do exist, assuming an owner is willing to follow through on the commitment made when the decision was first made to own a pet. It may cost

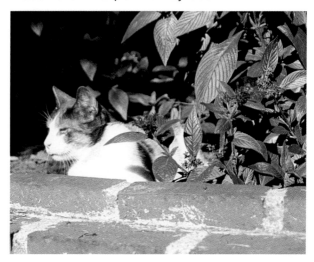

money and time, but that is part of the responsibility.

Where legitimate health reasons prompt the consideration of euthanasia, the cat's prognosis and quality of life are two parameters that affect such a decision. The term *prognosis* refers to the likelihood of a pet recovering from an injury, illness, or condition, or of it effectively responding to treatment efforts. Felines given a fair to excellent prognosis by a licensed veterinarian are certainly not candidates for euthanasia; they are candidates for treatment. If, on the other hand, the prognosis is poor to grave, then the second parameter—quality of life—comes into consideration. Those cats that are suffering from a terminal condition, yet still have the ability and desire to interact socially with their owners and to eat and drink on their own, can be assumed to have an acceptable quality of life. They should not be considered for euthanasia. However, for cats that do not meet these guidelines or for those that are experiencing moderate to severe pain on a continual basis—pain that cannot be effectively relieved without the use of extra-strength pain relievers— euthanasia should be strongly considered. If you ever are faced with such a decision, you will not be alone. Your veterinarian is trained in the euthanasia process and can be trusted to provide you with an accurate prognosis and quality-of-life assessment that will lead you to a correct decision.

One decision that should be made prior to euthanasia concerns the disposition of the remains following the procedure. Your veterinarian is knowledgeable about different options and can assist in you in making a decision regarding communal burial sites designated by your city or municipality, private burial sites, including pet memorial parks, or cremation. If you choose a mode of private burial, realize that most cities have laws restricting the burial of animals within city limits. Be sure to check your city code.

The decision for you to be with your pet at the time of euthanasia is strictly a matter of choice. If you choose not to be present, rest assured that your pet will experience the comfort and reassurance of gentle and caring hands during those final moments of its life. If you do elect to stay by your cat's side during the process, remain as calm as possible so as not to upset your pet. Gently stroke your cat's head, giving comfort and reassurance that the suffering will soon be over. Remember too, that few veterinarians take comfort in this task; veterinarians went to school to learn how to preserve life, not take it.

The only discomfort a pet may feel during the euthanasia process occurs with the initial insertion of the needle or catheter into the skin and vein. The administration and action of the euthanasia solution itself are painless. Depending upon the mental state and behavior of your pet or upon the degree of pain existing from an injury or illness, your veterinarian may administer a sedative to calm and relax the patient prior to administering the euthanasia solution. Once the euthanasia agent is injected, death takes only seconds. In rare instances, a vocalization or a heavy gasp may be heard as the agent is administered. In addition, evacuation of the bowels and urinary bladder can occur. Pet owners who insist on being present during the euthanasia procedure must realize that these occurrences are not associated with pain or discomfort in any way. Those portions of the brain responsible for conscious perception and pain are shut down long before the areas of the brain governing these responses are stimulated by the euthanasia solution. The pet experiences a peaceful, painless, and dignified death.

Once the euthanasia procedure is completed, don't hesitate to ask further questions and solicit input from your veterinarian if you are so inclined. Science and research have demonstrated that a strong bonding does occur between people and their pets. In fact, courses on this human-companion animal bond, the strength of which depends on numerous relationship factors, are taught in veterinary colleges across the country. The friendship a feline companion can provide is often difficult to duplicate. Losing such a friend can be quite traumatic, and it is important to realize that grieving is a perfectly natural and expected response to the loss of a pet. There is a stigma in our society about grieving openly for a pet that has died or has been put to sleep. However, failure to do so only causes a buildup of strong emotion and confusion. This is not only psychologically unhealthy, but as most doctors will point out, physically unhealthy as well. The more you understand about the grieving process and its four stages (denial, anger, depression, acceptance), the quicker the burden of your loss will be lifted. Many excellent books have been written on this subject, and they are readily available at your favorite bookstore or local library.

Pet loss support groups, which exist across the country, can help pet owners endure the loss of a beloved pet. These groups recognize the strength of the human-companion animal bond and understand its effects during such a difficult time, and that can be quite comforting to a grieving pet owner. To locate support groups near you, contact your veterinarian, the local or state veterinary medical association, the American Veterinary Medical Association, or a local veterinary college. Some veterinary schools have actual pet-loss counselors on staff ready to assist you in your time of need.

In addition to support groups, many psychologists and psychiatrists in private practice are well trained in pet loss grieving and support, and can be called upon to provide one-on-one counseling in such matters. You can usually obtain a

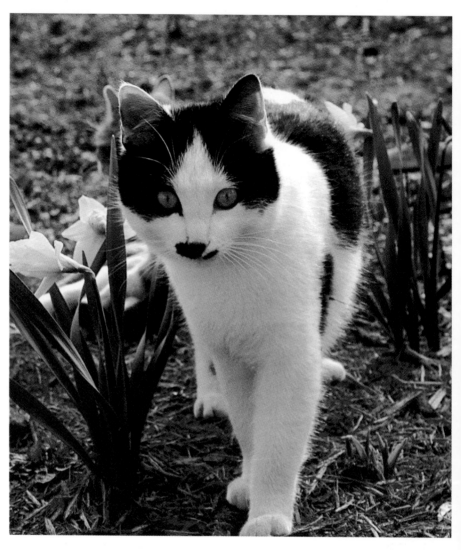

list of such specialists by contacting your local or state associations affiliated with these professions.

Donations made in memory of your pet are an excellent means by which you can preserve the precious memory of your faithful companion, and at the same time, help other pets still facing the trials of this life. Your local humane society, the local or state veterinary medical association, or the nearest veterinary college will be able to assist you in making the proper arrangements.

Glossary

Aberration: Alteration; abnormality.

Abscess: Defined pocket of pus on or within an organ or a tissue.

Acariasis: Infestation with mites.

ACTH: Hormone produced by the pituitary gland that serves to regulate steroid production by the adrenal glands.

Acute: Sudden, pronounced onset of clinical disease; short duration.

Addison's disease: Disease characterized by an insufficient production of steroid hormones by the adrenal glands.

Adenocarcinoma: Malignant tumor involving glandular structures.

Adenoma: Benign tumor involving glandular structures.

ADH: Antidiuretic hormone.

Adrenal glands: Endocrine glands located next to the kidneys that produce, among other things, steroid hormones.

Aerobic: Requiring oxygen for life or function.

Allergen: Substance capable of producing an allergic response.

Allergy: Exaggerated immune response to some foreign substance.

Alopecia: Hair loss.

ALT (alanine aminotransferase): Liver enzyme.

Anaphylactic reaction: Dramatic fall in blood pressure caused by a massive release of histamine and other chemicals within the body.

Anemia: Reduction in the number of red blood cells found within the body.

Anesthesia: Purposeful induction of unconsciousness.

Anorexia: Loss of appetite.

Antibiotic: Chemical substance capable of killing bacteria or preventing their replication.

Antibodies: Protein structures produced by cells of the immune system that assist in the destruction of foreign organisms and substances.

Antigen: Substances capable of eliciting an immune response.

Anti-inflammatory medications: Drugs designed to counteract the effects of inflammation. These include corticosteroids, as well as nonsteroidal drugs such as aspirin and acetaminophen.

Antimicrobial: Chemical or substance designed to kill or prevent replication of infectious organisms.

Arrhythmias: Abnormal heartbeats.

Arteries: Vessels that carry blood away from the heart.

Arthritis: Inflammation involving a joint .

Ascarids: Roundworms.

Ascites: Fluid accumulation within the abdominal cavity.

Astringent: Substance that has drying capabilities when applied to a surface.

Atrophy: Shrinking; wasting.

Autoimmune hemolytic anemia: Autoimmune disease characterized by the destruction of red blood cells within the body by the body's own immune system.

Beneficial nematodes: Organisms that, when applied to a yard, will help rid that area of flea larvae.

Biopsy: Act of taking an actual tissue sample from an organ or mass and after proper preparation, examining the tissue microscopically for identification or for the presence of disease.

Bone marrow: Tissue found within bone that contains the precursors of blood cells.

Bowels: Small and large intestines.

Cachexia: Weight loss with an overall wasting appearance.

Cancer: Malignant neoplasia that spreads into surrounding tissue.

Carcinogen: Substance or agent capable of producing neoplastic changes in cells.

Carcinoma: Cancer involving epithelial cells.

Cardiac output: Measure of the heart's ability to pump and circulate blood.

Cardiomyopathy: Degeneration of the muscle comprising the heart.

Cardiovascular: Pertaining to the heart and blood vessels.

Cartilage: Sturdy, flexible type of tissue that forms various structures within the body and covers joint surfaces.

Castration: Removal of the testicles.

Cataract: Disease or genetically induced opacity of the lens of the eye.

CBC: Complete blood count.

CEHC: Cystic endometrial hyperplasia complex.

Central nervous system: Brain and spinal cord.

Chemotherapy: Treatment of neoplasia utilizing chemicals or drugs.

Chronic: Slower, gradual onset of clinical disease; long duration.

Chylothorax: Presence of lymph within the chest cavity.

Cirrhosis: Disease characterized by the replacement of healthy tissue with scar tissue.

Coalesce: Combine; consolidate.

Colitis: Inflammation of the colon.

Commercially available: Available over-the-counter at pet stores, pet suppliers, or veterinary offices.

Congenital disease: Disease condition present, whether noticeable or not, at birth.

Coronavirus: Causative agent of FIP in cats.

Corticosteroids: Chemical compounds produced by the adrenal glands that exhibit a wide variety of functions within the body; *see* Glucocorticosteroids.

Cryotherapy: Treatment of neoplasia utilizing extremely cold temperatures to freeze tumor cells.

Cushing's disease: Disease characterized by an overproduction of steroid hormones by the adrenal glands.

Cytology: Diagnostic tool characterized by the microscopic examination and identification of cells taken from fluids, discharges, masses, and tumors.

Definitive diagnosis: Diagnosis that has been confirmed by physical examination or by specific diagnostic tests and procedures.

Dehydration: Condition in which the water level within the body is below that required for normal body functions.

Demarcation: Differentiate; discriminate.

Dermatitis: Inflammation of the skin.

Diagnosis: Identification of the underlying cause of a particular behavior or disease symptom.

DIC: Disseminated intravascular coagulation; formation of small blood clots throughout the body in response to shock or some disease condition.

Dietary indiscretion: Consumption of foodstuffs or substances that are not a normal component of a pet's diet.

Dip: Highly concentrated form of an insecticide.

Distemper: Feline panleukopenia; parvovirus.

Diuretic: Drug that mobilizes fluid out of the body by promoting urination.

Dysfunction: Abnormality in function.

ECG: Electrocardiogram; also EKG.

Edema: Fluid retention within the tissues.

Efficacy: Competence; efficiency.

Effusion: Escape of fluid into an open space or cavity.

Electrolyte: Molecules found within the body that are able to conduct an electrical current.

Electromyogram: Test used to assess electrical activity within muscle tissue.

Endocrine: Pertaining to glands and hormones within the body.

Endoscope: Instrument used to internally visualize hollow organs and body cavities.

Enzyme: Chemical substance that enhances and increases the speed of metabolic reactions within the body.

Etiology: Cause of a disease.

Exacerbate: Aggravate; intensify.

Exercise intolerance: Inability to physically exert without becoming weak or lethargic.

Exorbitant: Excessive; outrageous.

Feline infectious anemia: Anemia caused by parasitism of red blood cells; haemobartonellosis.

FeLV: Feline leukemia virus.

FIE: Feline ischemic encephalopathy.

FIP: Feline infectious peritonitis.

FIV: Feline immunodeficiency virus.

FURD: Feline upper respiratory disease.

FUS: Feline urologic syndrome.

Gastrointestinal: Pertaining to the stomach and intestines.

Giardiasis: Intestinal disease caused by a specific protozoal organism.

Gingivitis: Inflammation of the gums.

Glaucoma: Increase in fluid pressure within the eye.

Glucocorticosteroids: One particular class of corticosteroids that are useful in veterinary medicine for the alleviation of inflammation and itching in cats, as well as the prevention or counteraction of circulatory shock.

Granuloma: Firm mass created by inflammatory cells surrounding a foreign agent or substance.

Halitosis: Bad breath.

Hemoglobin: Molecule found within red blood cells that carries oxygen molecules.

Hemorrhage: Bleeding.

Hemostasis: Ability of the body to control internal or external bleeding.

Hemostatic pathway: Sequence of events that occurs within the body whenever it is called upon to control hemorrhage.

Hepatic: Pertaining to or acting on the liver.

Hernia: Protrusion of an organ or tissue through an unnatural opening.

Herpesvirus: Organism causing feline viral rhinotracheitis.

Hormone: Protein or steroid compound that regulates specific physical and chemical reactions within the body.

Husbandry: Caring for a pet, including feeding, housing, grooming, and preventive health care.

Hybrid vigor: Genetic vitality and strength in offspring resulting from the mating of two purebred cats of differing breeds.

Hydrophobia: Fear of water.

Hypertrophy: Enlargement; excessive growth.

Hypoallergenic: Produces very little allergic response.

Hypokalemia: Low blood potassium levels.

IBD: Inflammatory bowel disease.

Icterus: Jaundice.

Ictus: True seizure activity.

Idiopathic: Term used to describe any condition for which the cause is unknown.

Immunize: Act of stimulating an immune response.

Immunotherapy: Treatment of neoplasia utilizing immune system components.

Implement: Put into place; take action.

Inappetence: Loss of appetite.

Incapacitate: Disable; render useless.

Incontinence: Inability to willfully control bodily eliminations.

Inflammation: Bodily response to disease characterized by heat, redness, swelling, and pain.

Innocuous: Harmless; inoffensive.

Insect growth regulator: Chemical substance designed to prevent the maturation of immature forms of insects into adults.

Insulin: Hormone that regulates the uptake and utilization of glucose within the body.

Integumentary: Pertaining to the skin and associated structures.

Intravenous fluids: Special solutions similar to fluids normally found within the body; used in treatment to correct dehydration and maintain normal water balance within the body, and to stimulate cardiac function and blood circulation.

Isoflurane: Type of gas anesthesia commonly selected for use in older pets because of its favorable safety margin.

Keratitis: Inflammation of the cornea.

Ketones: By-products of fat metabolism within the body.

Larva: Immature form of an insect.

Lenticular sclerosis: Cloudiness of the eye lenses occurring as a normal aging change in older cats.

Lethargy: Apathy; listlessness.

Leukocyte: White blood cell.

LSA: Lymphosarcoma.

Lumen: Interior of a hollow organ or structure.

Lupus: Autoimmune disease affecting the skin, mucous membranes, and various organs of the body.

Lymph: Liquid substance within the body. Contains immune cells, proteins, and fat molecules.

Lymphocyte: Type of white blood cell, some of which are capable of producing antibodies.

Malaise: Despondency; weakness.

Malignant: Type of tumor experiencing frenzied, uncontrolled growth or spread.

Mange: Infestation with mites.

Metabolism: Sum of all chemical reactions occurring within the body.

Metastasis: Spread of tumor cells from their site of origin to other parts of the body.

Metritis: Inflammation of the uterus.

Microencapsulation: Process by which chemicals, particularly insecticides, are treated to create a slow, timely, and consistent release when applied to the pet or environment.

Musculoskeletal: Pertaining to muscles, bones, and joints.

Myoglobin: Molecule found within muscle cells that binds oxygen.

Myopathy: Degenerative disease of muscle.

Myositis: Inflammation of muscle tissue.

Neoplasia: Abnormal division and growth of cells within the body.

Neuter: Removal of the ovaries and uterus in the female cat (ovariohysterectomy; spay) or testicles in the male (castration).

Nidus: Localized area of involvement; source.

Nodular: Round; protruding.

Noxious: Unpleasant; adverse.

Obesity: Disease condition in which excessive amounts of fat exist within the body.

Ophthalmic: Pertaining to the eyes.

Organophosphate: Extremely potent (and potentially toxic) class of chemical used in many insecticide products designed for flea and tick control in cats.

Otitis: Inflammation involving the ear.

Palatability: Taste and flavor appeal of a food.

Palliative: Alleviation of symptoms without curing.

Palpation: Diagnostic technique used by veterinarians that involves probing and touching of a particular region of the body using the hands and fingers.

Pancreatitis: Inflammation of the pancreas.

Parathyroid glands: Glands closely associated with the thyroid glands in cats and responsible for regulating levels of calcium within the body.

Parvovirus: Infectious organism that can strike the gastrointestinal system of cats and cause serious disease (feline panleukopenia).

Pemphigus: Autoimmune skin disease.

Perineal: Pertaining to the perineum.

Perineum: Region of the body located between the sexual organs and the anus.

Periodontal disease: Tooth and gum disease.

pH: Measurement used to express the acidity or alkalinity of a solution.

Physiologic: Pertaining to the body, its components, and their functioning.

Pituitary gland: Gland at the base of the brain. Produces and stores hormones, most of which control the release of other hormones throughout the body.

Platelet: Blood component that assists in the formation of blood clots.

Pneumothorax: Presence of air within the chest cavity (outside the lungs).

Polydipsia: Increased water consumption.

Polyphagia: Increased appetite.

Polyuria: Increased production and excretion of urine.

Progesterone: Sex hormone responsible for maintaining pregnancy in the female.

Proliferation: Growth; enlargement; reproduction.

Puberty: Age of sexual maturity.

PVD: Peripheral vestibular disorder.

Pyometra: Condition characterized by pus- or fluid-filled uterus.

Pyothorax: Presence of pus within the chest cavity.

Pyrethrin: Relatively safe chemical used in many flea and tick control products.

Rabies: Uniformly fatal viral disease transmitted primarily by the saliva from infected animals.

Radiograph: Pictorial representation of a structure or region of the body created by placing that structure or region over special photographic film and then passing X rays through it.

Regenerative anemia: Anemic condition in which the body is actively replacing those red blood cells that are lost.

Residual: Long-acting; prolonged effects.

Rhinitis: Inflammation of the nasal passages.

Sanguineous: Blood-tinged fluid.

Sarcoma: Malignant neoplasia originating from connective tissue within the body.

Sebaceous gland: Gland that

secretes sebum and is attached to a hair follicle.

Seborrhea: Condition characterized by an abnormal production of skin keratin, causing the skin to crust and scale.

Sebum: Oily secretion produced by specialized skin glands.

Sedative: Chemical agent that, when administered to a pet, exerts a calming and relaxing effect that is useful for restraint and minor diagnostic and treatment procedures.

Sensory: Pertaining to vision, hearing, touch, taste, and smell.

Shock (circulatory shock): Life-threatening condition characterized by a gradual shutdown of vital body processes, including blood circulation.

Spay: Removal of the ovaries and uterus in the female cat.

Sphincter: Muscular band of tissue designed to regulate the entrance into or exit from an organ.

Stomatitis: Inflammation and infection involving the mouth.

Subcutaneous: Beneath the skin.

Supplement: Add; enhance.

Symmetry: Balance; congruity.

Syncope: Loss of consciousness caused by oxygen deprivation to the brain.

Systemic: Acting internally; within the body.

Taurine: Essential amino acid in cats; deficiencies can lead to cardiomyopathy and retinal degeneration.

Tenesmus: Straining to defecate.

Tentative diagnosis: An unconfirmed diagnosis that is usually based upon history, clinical signs, physical examination, and preliminary laboratory findings.

Thoracic: Pertaining to the thorax (chest cavity).

Thrombocytopenia: Abnormally low number of platelets within the blood.

Thromboembolism: Blood clot blocking the flow of blood through an artery.

Tracheobronchitis: Inflammation of the trachea and bronchi.

Ulcer: Erosion in the lining or surface of an organ.

Ultrasound: Utilization of sound waves passed through the body to create a picture of internal organs and structures on a special screen.

Urethra: Tubelike organ that carries urine from the bladder to the exterior of the body.

Uroliths: Mineralized stones found within the urinary tract.

Vaccine: Man-made preparation of antigenic substances designed to elicit an immune response when introduced into the body.

Veins: Vessels that carry blood back to the heart.

Vertebrae: Bones comprising the spinal column, through which the spinal cord passes.

Vitamins: Organic substances needed for many physiologic processes within the body.

Vitamin K: Vitamin that plays an important role in hemostasis.

X ray: Type of radiation used to obtain a radiograph.

Index